# Epidural Administration - New Perspectives and Uses

*Edited by Sotonye Fyneface-Ogan*

Published in London, United Kingdom

Epidural Administration - New Perspectives and Uses
http://dx.doi.org/10.5772/intechopen.105323
Edited by Sotonye Fyneface-Ogan

Contributors
Prashanth Jagadeesha Prabhu, Chimaobi Tim Nnaji, José Correa, Henry Cortes, Lucia Correa, Rita López, Allison Kalstein Apple, Joel Yarmush, Sangeetha Kamath, Sangeetha Setty, Vandana Gupta, Prabhdeep Singh, Sotonye Fyneface-Ogan, Fiekabo Ogan-Hart, Katarina Tomulić Brusich, Lara Valenčić, Željka Polonijo, Kingsley U. Tobi



First published in London, United Kingdom, 2023 by IntechOpen
IntechOpen is the global imprint of INTECHOPEN LIMITED, registered in England and Wales, registration number: 11086078, 5 Princes Gate Court, London, SW7 2QJ, United Kingdom

British Library Cataloguing-in-Publication Data
A catalogue record for this book is available from the British Library

Additional hard and PDF copies can be obtained from orders@intechopen.com

Epidural Administration - New Perspectives and Uses
Edited by Sotonye Fyneface-Ogan
p. cm.
Print ISBN 978-1-83768-417-5
Online ISBN 978-1-83768-418-2
eBook (PDF) ISBN 978-1-83768-419-9

# Meet the editor

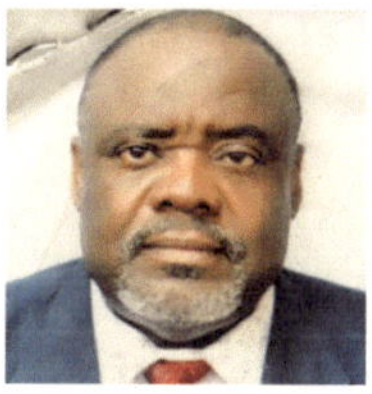

Sotonye Fyneface-Ogan is a teacher and pioneering researcher in the field of obstetric anaesthesiology with a special interest in the epidural space and its uses. He is a professor of obstetric anaesthesiology and a lecturer at the Faculty of Clinical Sciences of the University of Port Harcourt, Nigeria. Currently, Prof. Fyneface-Ogan heads the Obstetric Anaesthesia Unit of the University of Port Harcourt Teaching Hospital. He is a senior examiner in the Faculty of Anaesthesia, West African College of Surgeons, and a trainer in obstetric anaesthesia for the World Federation of Societies of Anaesthesiologists.

# Contents


**Preface** **IX**

**Section 1**
Identification of the Epidural Space **1**

**Chapter 1** **3**
Perspective Chapter: Epidural Administration – Various Advances in Techniques
*by Sotonye Fyneface-Ogan and Fiekabo Ogan-Hart*

**Chapter 2** **15**
Epidural: Loss of Resistance
*by Prashanth Jagadeesha Prabhu*

**Section 2**
Pharmacology of Epidural Medications **35**

**Chapter 3** **37**
Physiology and Pharmacology of Epidurally Administered Drugs
*by Katarina Tomulić Brusich, Lara Valenčić and Željka Polonijo*

**Chapter 4** **77**
Perspective Chapter: Epidural Administration – New Perspectives and Uses
*by Allison Kalstein Apple, Sangeetha Kamath, Joel Yarmush, Sangeetha Setty, Vandana Gupta and Prabhdeep Singh*

**Section 3**
Epidural Administration and Cell-Based Therapy **95**

**Chapter 5** **97**
Perspectives of Cell-Based Therapy for Degenerative Diseases of the Spine: The Reason for Choosing the Epidural Space
*by José Correa, Henry Cortés, Lucia Correa and Rita López*

**Section 4**
Epidural Administration and the ICU **113**

**Chapter 6** **115**
Epidural Analgesia for Pain Management in the Intensive Care Unit
*by Kingsley U. Tobi*

**Section 5**
Epidural Service and Low Resource Setting **125**

**Chapter 7** **127**
Perspective Chapter: Epidural Anaesthesia Service Delivery in Anaesthesia Workforce Constrained Regions
*by Chimaobi Tim Nnaji*

# Preface

The epidural space around the spinal cord is one of the most explored and exploited spaces in human anatomy. The last two decades have seen an exponential increase in the use of the epidural space to administer medications to enhance anaesthesia and analgesia, opening a new horizon in the management of patients in clinical settings.

*Epidural Administration - New Perspectives and Uses* focuses on recent advances in the exploration and exploitation of this space. The first chapter of this unique book reviews the various ways of achieving epidural administration of agents into the epidural space. Chapter 2 describes the loss of resistance (LOR) technique, the preferred method for identifying the epidural space, and explains how a sudden change in resistance is detected with the passage of the epidural needle tip from the ligamentum flavum into the epidural space. The third chapter provides insight into this complex and comprehensive topic to demonstrate a predictable pattern that can provide a safe and accurate guide to clinical practice. Chapter 3 also highlights the many factors that have an impact on drug physiology and pharmacology in the epidural space, and discusses how epidural anaesthesia or the expected effect of another medication can be modified.

Chapter 4 covers basic anatomical considerations, general and obstetric physiology, epidural techniques and position, the use of ultrasound for epidural placement, pharmacological drugs used in epidurals, complementary and supplementary regional blocks with epidurals, other remedies when epidurals are not viable or fail, and local anesthesia systemic toxicity. Chapter 5 discusses lumbar disc degeneration as a common progressive, chronic disorder and a major cause of low back pain. The authors show that epidural platelet-rich plasma injections can cause a significant release of growth factors to improve the healing of wounds and the processes of tissue regeneration, and in the treatment of cellular involution that takes place with aging.

Adequate pain control in the intensive care unit (ICU) is essential and adds to optimal patient care with improved outcomes. However, epidural administration of opioids is rarely considered in patients in ICU experiencing significant pain. Chapter 6 describes how epidural administration of various analgesics can be used to manage the pain experienced by these critically ill patients. Chapter 7 highlights the importance of human, technical and economic resources as prerequisites for effective epidural services. It suggests ways of tackling the constraints experienced in low- and middle-income countries.

The chapters in this book are well-written by authors with in-depth knowledge of the topics. The book will be a good armamentarium for all anaesthetists in clinical practice.

**Sotonye Fyneface-Ogan**
Professor,
Obstetric Anaesthesia Unit,
University of Port Harcourt Teaching Hospital,
Port Harcourt, Nigeria

Section 1

# Identification of the Epidural Space

Chapter 1

# Perspective Chapter: Epidural Administration – Various Advances in Techniques

*Sotonye Fyneface-Ogan and Fiekabo Ogan-Hart*


## Abstract

First described by Fidel Pages in 1921, epidural administration is a technique in which a medicine is injected into the epidural space has undergone various modifications and approaches in recent years. Epidural administration also involves the placement of a catheter into the epidural space, which may remain in place for the duration of the treatment. These advances have changed the face of clinical practice and improved the patient management. Modification to the approach of epidural administration has moved from the single-shot epidural administration to programmed injections. The use of these improved techniques has reduced complications associated with epidural administration and improved care. The administration of medication into this space has been considered as safe and effective for providing pain relief during childbirth and surgery. A review of these modes of administration will highlight the importance of each of the techniques.


**Keywords:** epidural administration, techniques, epidural analgesia, epidural catheter, epidural space

## 1. Introduction

Epidural administration of medications has been used in many surgical and anesthetic managements of patients. It is currently mostly used for postoperative management in the regions of the body amenable to it [1]. It has a wide margin of safety in experienced hands. Beyond its use in postoperative pain management, it has been indicated in the administration of steroids, contrast agents and many others.

It is important to know that the positioning of the patients requiring epidural administration is determined by patient's comfort, compliance and preference of the attending. Insertion of the needle is commonly performed in either sitting, or flexed lateral position, although the sitting position has higher rate of first pass insertion and shorter duration (skin puncture to correct needle placement time) [2].

This chapter will review the various methods epidural administration of agents into the epidural space can be achieved.

## 2. Methods of identifying epidural space

Epidural administration of pharmacologically active agents would be impossible without proper identification of the space. This is most frequent cause of failed epidural administration [3]. Patient positioning, the use of a midline or paramedian approach, and the method used for catheter fixation can all influence the success rate.

For epidural injection using the midline approach to be successful, the Tuohy needle would have to traverse the skin, subcutaneous fat, supraspinous ligament, interspinous ligament, ligamentum flavum, and then into the epidural space. The epidural space is a potential space, the loss of resistance on a plunger is indicative of the entrance to the epidural space. Localization of the space is one of the major key steps in epidural administration. Many ingenious devices have been designed to improve the success of the puncture procedure and are based on the principle of loss of resistance within the epidural space.

## 3. Epidural space identification methods

1. Ogan's slingshot epidural syringe: This simple device uses a rubber sling mounted on the plunger of the syringe which generates a head pressure on the plunger (**Figure 1**) [4].

   With a mounted Tuohy needle advancing into the epidural space, the plunger collapses as the needle gets into the epidural space. This device which depends on loss of resistance to air gives about 95-97% accuracy in identifying the epidural space.

2. Epidural balloon: This is also a device which depends on the negative pressure exhibited by the denting of the ligamentum flavum during penetration of the Tuohy needle (**Figure 2**).

   The balloon attached to plastic device collapses (or the air in the balloon is sucked in) as the needle enters into the epidural space.

3. Episure™ AutoDetect syringe: This is another epidural space localization device (**Figure 3**).

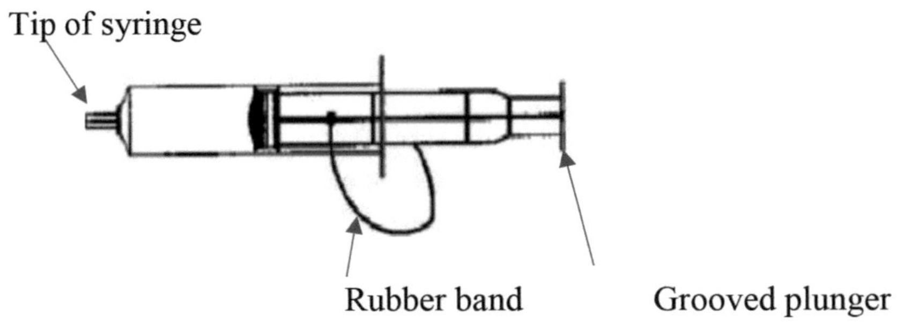


**Figure 1.**
*Slingshot® epidural syringe.*

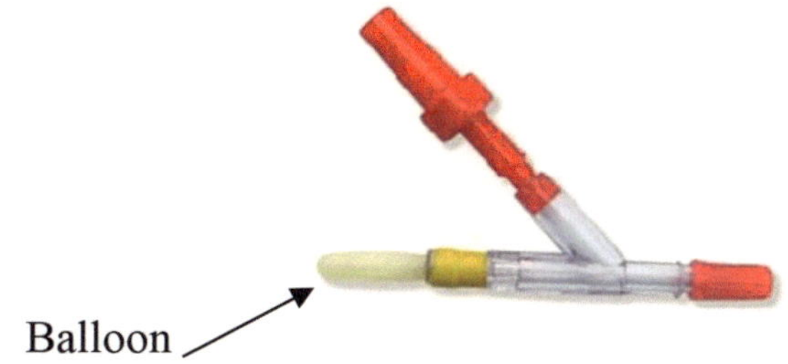


**Figure 2.**
*Epidural balloon – Vygon© UK.*

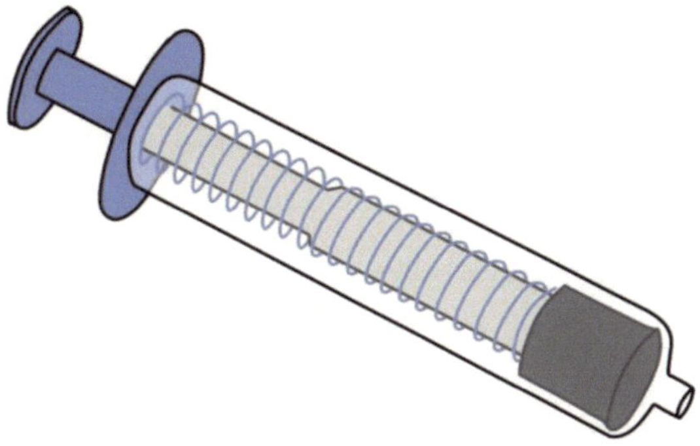

**Figure 3.**
*Episure™ syringe.*

This device works better when it is filled with normal saline and with an advancing mounted Tuohy needle into the space the plunger automatically loses resistance, which "provides an objective, visual confirmation that the epidural space has been identified." Other devices used in the identifying the epidural space include the use of ultrasound guide [5], spring-loaded syringes, episure [6].

4. Epidrum©: This device depends on a low pressure loss of resistance to facilitate epidural space identification. The device is fixed between the syringe and needle and, filled with air to inflate its diaphragm. As the needle advances and gets into the epidural space, there will be a visible collapse of the diaphragm marking the endpoint of space identification. One great advantage of this device is that, it allows a slow advancement of the needle with both hands making a more accurate space identification possible (**Figure 4**).

   When inflated and connected to the Tuohy needle, Epidrum allows higher pressure changes due to the location of the epidural space to be differentiated from those due to smaller changes in the path through the different tissues of the patient [7].

5. EpiFaith© syringe: EpiFaith is a relatively new device used in identifying the epidural space by loss of resistance technique. When the operator attaches the syringe to the Tuohy needle, the spring is held in place by the locking mechanism (where the yellow ring on the piston meets the blue plunger). The operator then pushes the syringe plunger forward to engage the spring. The operator can now

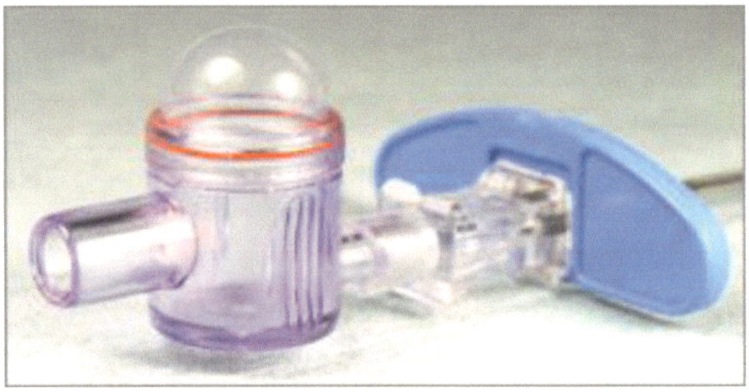

**Figure 4.**
*Epidrum©.*

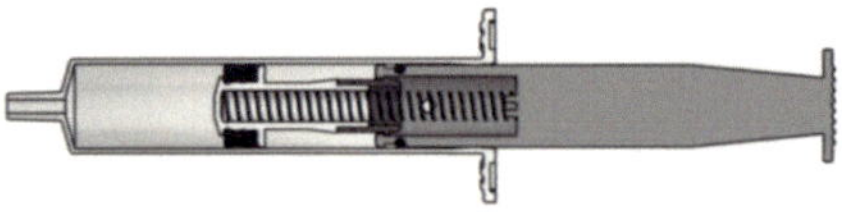

**Figure 5.**
*EpiFaith© syringe (drawing provided by flat medical Inc. (Taipei City, Taiwan)).*

advance the needle with two hands braced against the back. When the Tuohy needle tip enters the epidural space and there is a loss of resistance, the piston advances, and the yellow is visible. The piston moving forward, and the appearance of the yellow color are indicators of a loss of resistance [8] (**Figure 5**).

It is a device that ensures the Touhy needles comes to an abrupt halt with the pressure change in the epidural space. EpiFaith is mechanically driven and reduces the risk of accidental dural puncture.

6. Acoustic puncture assist device: Failure in identifying the epidural space could be a great challenge to the attending Anesthetist. One way of correct identification is the use of Acoustic puncture assist device [9]. This method is designed to detect and signal by tone, the loss of resistance encountered during epidural procedure. The device records the pressure changes during epidural puncture of the ligamentum flavum. When in use, it provides an objective, visible pressure readings which again help in identifying the epidural space.

7. Fiber Bragg sensors: The mechanism of action of this device is characterized by periodic modulation of the refraction index along the axis of the fiber core. An abrupt relaxation of the fiber is observed as it passes from a thin and very hard tissue (like the ligament flavum) to a soft region (epidural space) signaling the entrance into the epidural space. This form of epidural space identification is still being researched in humans [10].

8. Ultrasound scan: Using either the linear or curved probe, the ultrasound can be used to guide the needle in identifying the epidural space. It is well known to provide a real time reliable information about the surrounding tissues when traversing to enter the epidural space. It has been associated with a high success rate.

*DOI: http://dx.doi.org/10.5772/intechopen.108642*

While most of the methods described earlier depend on loss of resistance to air (which could introduce air to cause patchy blocks), Evron et al. demonstrated the relevance of loss of resistance to lidocaine which could best be described as loss of resistance to fluid [11]. The advantage of Evron et al. technique added more value in which dilutional factor with saline is circumvented rather synergistic to other local anesthetics administered into the epidural space.

## 4. Methods of epidural administration

Various methods have been advanced in carrying out epidural administration in clinical practice. Each of these methods is unique in its own way. The purpose of epidural administration could be short term or long term; depending on the need of the patient or the purpose for which it is administered. Epidural administration of medications can be effected through:

a. Manual (bolus) injection

b. Delivered by a machine

- Volumetric epidural infusion
- Epidural syringe pump

There are ways in which the administration can be conducted:

i. Single bolus injection

ii. Intermittent bolus injection

iii. Continuous injection

### 4.1 Single shot epidural administration (SSEA)

Single shot epidural injections, involves injecting a single dose of a drug. It eliminates the risk associated with epidural infusion through an indwelling catheter, such as restricting mobility limited options for anticoagulant therapy, injections and also for steroid injections. It is frequently used in management of radiculopathies [12]. This technique does not require the retention of an epidural catheter. While single-shot epidural administration may be ideal in some settings, the incidence of complications has been argued to be the same with the use of continuous epidural with use of a catheter. However its application is well out of place in modern labor analgesia practice. It is quite difficult to accurately quantify and qualify the adequacy of sensory level of analgesia following a single-shot. The use of a single-shot is in favor of epidural administration of steroids for radicular pain and others [13].

### 4.2 Continuous epidural administration (CEA)

Continuous epidural administration can be carried out with the use of either a volumetric pump or syringe pump. Each of these devices works differently. While the volumetric pump allows a calculated dose of medication in an infusion bag to flow through the epidural catheter at a predetermined rate, the syringe pump delivers a calculated dose of medication through a syringe and catheter at predetermined rate to the patient. Continuous epidural infusions offer a safety advantage over intermittent epidural injections because peak and trough levels of the analgesic agent are avoided.

Continuous epidural analgesia is commonly used for labor analgesia, postoperative pain control after thoracic, abdominal, lower extremity, and rarely, upper extremity surgeries. An infusion pump can be used to carry out epidural administration of medications. This device is commonly used in areas such as obstetrics to deliver medications (e.g., bupivacaine or other controlled substances) for maintenance of analgesia during labor.

### *4.2.1 Infusion or volumetric pump*

This plays an important role in postoperative pain relief. It requires repeated injections or continuous infusion of local anesthetic solutions, using a volumetric pump, capable of delivering continuous and very specific amounts of fluid at either a slow or fast rate, with the presence of an indwelling catheter. The initial dose establishes the extent of analgesia and continuous infusion preserves it. It is associated with the risk of misplacing the catheter and infection [14]. However, a primary safety concern with epidural volumetric infusion pump is the risk of delivery through an incorrect

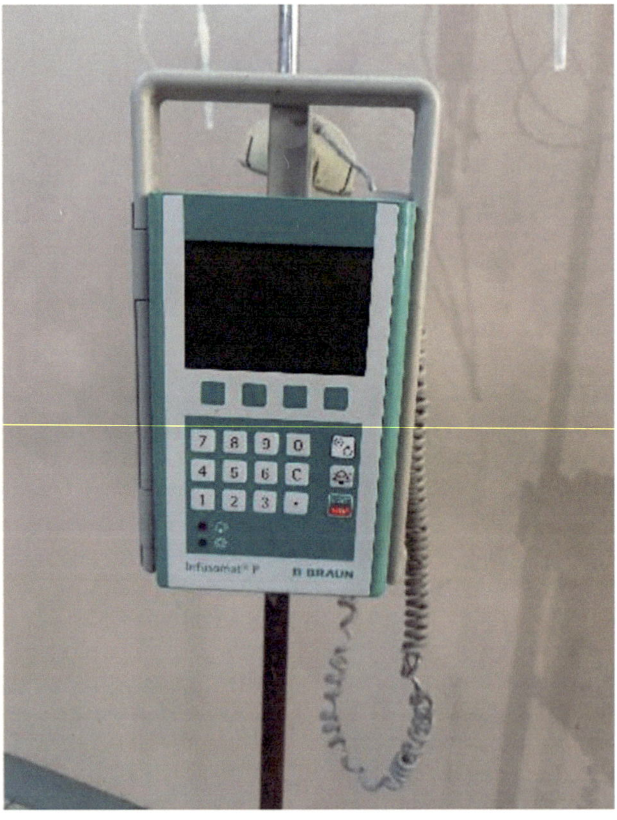


**Figure 6.**
*A volumetric pump - Infusomat® P (B Braun).*

route of administration, which can happen when epidural infusions are mixed with intravenous infusions. Infusing medications intended for epidural delivery through intravenous sites or vice versa can be detrimental (**Figure 6**).

#### *4.2.2 Syringe pump*

The syringe pump can be used to deliver a calculated dose and rate of a medication into the epidural space through an epidural catheter (**Figure 7**).

The pump maintains a steady stream of flow of the medication administered without the patient's input.

### 4.3 Combine spinal epidural administration (CSEA)

Epidural administration can be achieved through the use of a combined spinal epidural technique. The epidural component of this procedure is through the placement of catheter into the epidural space [15]. The medications to be administered can be done through the use of an infusion (volumetric) or syringe pump.

### 4.4 Patient controlled epidural administration (PCEA)

The patient-controlled epidural analgesia (PCEA) technique has been recently set up as a preferred mode of epidural drug delivery and used widely. The development of PCEA allows patients to superimpose a limited volume of bolus dosing on an already established continuous infusion (**Figure 8**).

It has been found that patients with PCEA require less local anesthetic than patients with continuous epidural administration, to achieve a similar quality of epidural analgesia [16]. To forestall overdosing, the patient controlled pump is incorporated with a lockout mechanism which prevents repeated self-dosing within a given time interval.

### 4.5 Computer integrated patient-controlled epidural injection (CIPCEA)

Computer-integrated patient-controlled epidural analgesia (CIPCEA) is a novel epidural delivery system programmed to analyze the pharmacologic agent use across the last hour and adjusts the background infusion rate according to an algorithm [17] (**Figure 9**).

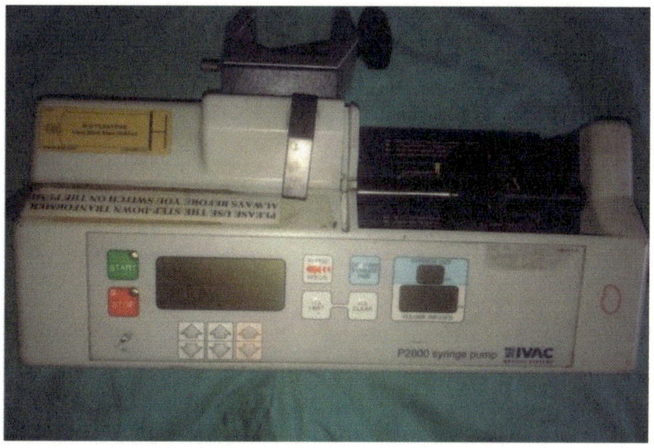


**Figure 7.**
*P2000 syringe pump (IVAC®).*

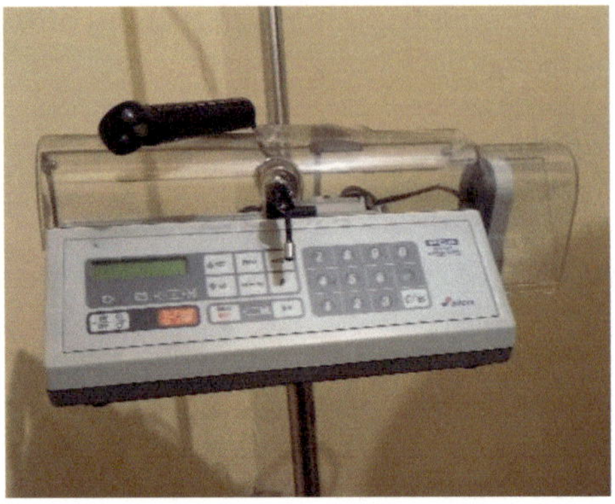

**Figure 8.**
*Patient-controlled syringe pump SP-14S (aitecs©).*

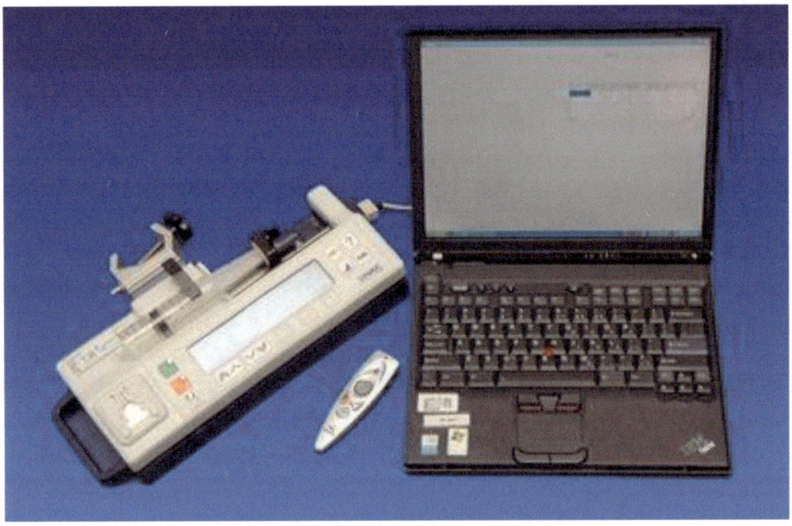

**Figure 9.**
*Computer integrated patient controlled epidural pump (first generation computer integrated infusion pump set-up using an IBM Thinkpad laptop (IBM, USA) connected to a modified syringe pump (IVAC P700, Alaris, UK).*

This novel method of epidural drug injection automatically adjusts the injection rates based on the patients need for analgesia [18]. When compared with the conventional patient controlled injection, there was more patient satisfaction and less local anesthesia use in the CIPCEI group [18].

### 4.6 Programmed intermittent bolus epidural injection (PIEBA)

Programmed intermittent epidural bolus (PIEB) is a new way of injecting local anesthetic agents into the epidural space through an epidural catheter at fixed time intervals [19].

This is an automated method of administering boluses of local anesthetic solution into the epidural space at fixed time intervals. It has been described as a method that works perfectly well with patient-controlled epidural administration (PCEA) [16].

The combination of methods prolongs the duration of analgesia, reduces motor block, lowers incidence of breakthrough pain, and reduces local anesthetic consumption compared to continuous epidural injection [20]. However, it remains unclear what is the optimal PIEBA dosing regimen.

## 5. Conclusion

Epidural administration is a valuable tool in clinical practice. It has been used in various management or treatment of pain such as postoperative, labor analgesia, steroid administration, injection of platelet-rich plasma concentrate and other needs in clinical medicine. More researches are still on in exploring other ways the epidural space can be beneficial in clinical practice.

## Author details

Sotonye Fyneface-Ogan* and Fiekabo Ogan-Hart
Obstetric Anaesthesia Unit, University of Port Harcourt Teaching Hospital, Port Harcourt, Nigeria

*Address all correspondence to: soglonye@yahoo.com

## References

[1] Avila Hernandez AN, Singh P. Epidural Anesthesia. Treasure Island (FL): StatPearls Publishing; 2022. p. 2022

[2] Nishi M, Usukaura A, Kidani Y, et al. Which is a better position for insertion of a high thoracic epidural catheter: Sitting or lateral decubitus? Journal of Cardiothoracic and Vascular Anesthesia. 2006;**20**(5):656-658

[3] Hermanides J, Hollmann MW, Stevens MF, Lirk P. Failed epidural: Causes and management. British Journal of Anaesthesia. 2012;**109**(2):144-154

[4] Fyneface-Ogan S. Epidural space localization: A novel a slingshot approach. African Journal of Anesthesia and Intensive Care. 2014;**14**:1-5

[5] Fyneface-Ogan S, Mato CN. A clinical experience with epidural balloon in the localisation of the epidural space in labouring parturients. Nigerian Quarterly Journal of Hospital Medicine. 2008;**18**:166-169

[6] Riley ET, Carvalho B. The Episure™ syringe: A novel loss of resistance syringe for locating the epidural space. Anesthesia and Analgesia. 2007;**105**:1164-1166

[7] Sawada A, Kii N, Yoshikawa Y, Yamakage M. Epidrum(®): A new device to identify the epidural space with an epidural Tuohy needle. Journal of Anesthesia. 2012;**26**(2):292-295

[8] Athar MW, Guo N, Ortner C, Carvalho B, Abir G, Riley ET. An observational pilot study of a novel loss of resistance syringe for locating the epidural space. International Journal of Obstetric Anesthesia. 2021;**47**:102984. DOI: 10.1016/j.ijoa.2021.102984

[9] Lechner TJ, van Wijk MG, Maas AJ, van Dorsten FR, Drost RA, Langenberg CJ, et al. Clinical results with the acoustic puncture assist device, a new acoustic device to identify the epidural space. Anesthesia and Analgesia. 2003;**96**:1183-1187

[10] Carotenuto B, Micco A, Ricciardi A, Amorizzo E, Mercieri M, Cutolo A, et al. Optical guidance systems for epidural space identification. IEEE Journal of Selected Topics in Quantum Electronics. 2017;**23**:371-379

[11] Evron S, Sessler D, Sadan O. Identification of the epidural space: Loss of resistance with air, lidocaine, or the combination of air and lidocaine. Anesthesia and Analgesia. 2004;**99**:245-250

[12] Todorov L, Vadeboncouer T. Etiology and use of "hanging drop" technique: A review. Pain Research and Treatment. 2014;**2014**:146750. DOI: 10.1155/2014/146750

[13] Patel K, Chopra P, Upadhyayula S. Epidural Steroid Injections. Treasure Island (FL): StatPearls Publishing; 2022

[14] Elsharkawy H, Sonny A, Chin KJ. Localisation of epidural space; a review of available technologies. Journal of Anaesthesiology Clinical Pharmacology. 2017;**33**(1):16-27

[15] Ueda K, Ueda W, Manabe M. A comparative study of sequential epidural bolus technique and continuous epidural bolus technique and continuous epidural infusion. Anaesth. 2005;**103**(1):126-129

[16] Sng BL, Woo D, Leong WL, Wang H, Assam PN, Sia AT. Comparison

of computer-integrated patient-controlled epidural analgesia with no initial basal infusion versus moderate basal infusion for labor and delivery: A randomized controlled trial. Journal of Anaesthesiology Clinical Pharmacology. 2014;**30**:496-501

[17] Lim Y, Sia AT, Ocampo CE. Comparison of computer integrated patient controlled epidural analgesia vs. conventional patient controlled epidural analgesia for pain relief in labour. Anaesthesia. 2006;**61**(4):339-344

[18] Kim YJ, Lee DK, Kwon HJ, et al. Programmed intermittent epidural bolus versus continuous epidural infusion in major upper abdominal surgery: A retrospective comparative study. Journal of Clinical Medicine. 2021;**10**:5382. DOI: 10.3390/jcm10225382

[19] Wang LY, Wu ZH, Hu LJ, et al. Programmed intermittent epidural bolus for post-cesarean delivery analgesia: A randomized controlled double-blind trial. Journal of Anesthesia. 2022;**36**(1):32-37. DOI: 10.1007/s00540-021-03002-x

[20] George RB, Allen TK, Habib AS. Intermittent epidural bolus compared with continuous epidural infusions for labour analgesia: A systematic review and meta-analysis. Anaesthesia & Analgesia. 2013;**116**(1):133-144

Chapter 2

# Epidural: Loss of Resistance

*Prashanth Jagadeesha Prabhu*

## Abstract

The epidural space is present above the dura also called as extradural space. This space contains spinal nerve roots and other contents with Batson's venous plexus. The lumbar epidural space is more than atmospheric pressure. Hence, one of the hypothesis for loss of resistance (LOR) during epidural is the loss of pressure exerted by dense ligamentum flavum. There are many methods to find the loss of resistance (LOR) technique. Two most common methods followed are loss of air technique and loss of saline technique. The recent advances speak about epidural waveform analysis for correct position of epidural catheter which is helpful in labor analgesia.

**Keywords:** epidural, loss of resistance, saline, air, methods, pressure

## 1. Introduction

The epidural needle (also known as extradural space or peridural space) pierces the skin, subcutaneous tissue, supraspinous ligament, interspinous ligament, ligamentum flavum, and finally epidural space (EDS). The failure rate of lumbar epidural is 27% and thoracic epidural is 32% [1].

## 2. History of origin of loss of resistance to epidural space

In 1921, Sicard and Forestier described loss of resistance (LOR) using lipiodol. Lipiodol is a chemical compound with 40% iodine with vegetable oil or poppy seed oil [2].

In 1928, Heldt and Moloney attempted to check the epidural pressure with spinal puncture needle with stopcock. They attached the manometer to the stopcock to measure the pressure. A negative pressure of −1 to −18 mm of mercury was recorded by the manometer once the needle was pushed deeper to the ligamentum flavum [3].

## 3. Different methods available for the loss of resistance

Various methods are described for epidural loss of resistance.

### 3.1 Classification based on type of sensation appreciated

Three categories of LOR have been described as:

- tactile end point (loss of resistance),
- visual end point (negative pressure recognition), and
- auditory end point (acoustic fall in tonal pitch) [4].

The other classification of various methods to identify EDS (epidural space).

### 3.2 Based on level or position of needle and epidural space

Three categories are described:

- Needle before entering the epidural space or guiding the needle to EDS,
- Needle during entry into epidural space or identifying entry into the EDS, and
- Post needle entry into epidural space or confirming needle/catheter location in the EDS [5].

Guiding the needle to EDS.

- Ultrasound-guided techniques
- Needle tracking methods
- Guidance positioning system for regional anesthesia (SonixGPS)
- Real-time 3D/4D ultrasonography
- Ultrasound imaging with pre-acquired three-dimensional images of spine
- Ultrasound through needle
- Needle through ultrasound
- Machine vision
- Acoustic radiation force impulse (ARFI) imaging
- Fluoroscopy

Identifying entry into epidural space (modifications of the loss of resistance technique).

- Membrane in syringe technique
- Epidural balloon
- Epidrum

- Episure Autodetect
- Auditory and visual display of pressure wave
- Bioimpedance
- Optical reflectance spectroscopy
- Optical coherence tomography (OCT)

Confirm catheter location in epidural space.

- Epidural stimulation test
- Electrocardiography (ECG)-guided system
- Epidurography
- Epidural pressure waveform analysis
- Near-infrared tracking system
- Ultrasound

### 3.3 The detection of epidural space can also be classified as two types: Subjective and objective types

The subjective type can be subdivided into two types—human-based subjective type and equipment-based subjective type.

The objective type can be subdivided into two types—equipment-based objective type and ultrasound-based objective type.

#### *3.3.1 Human-based subjective type epidural space detection*

1. Loss of air
2. Loss of fluid
3. Saline with air bubble
4. Lidocaine
5. KSMM (the combined plunger pressure—manometer method)
6. BiP (Bidigital Pressure) test
7. Use of hanging drop
8. Cerebral spinal fluid (CSF) ceased to drip

9. Sterile water injection
10. Loss of guidewire resistance (LOGR, epidural space finder)
11. Membrane in syringe technique
12. Epidural Queckenstedt test
13. Cold test
14. Hissing sound
15. Second needle method

*3.3.2 Equipment-based subjective-type epidural space detection*

1. Acoustic puncture assist device (APAD)
2. LOR syringe with fluoroscopy
3. EpiFaith syringe
4. Episure autodetect syringe
5. Epidrum
6. Epidural balloon
7. Electrocardiography (ECG)-guided system
8. Drip infusion method

*3.3.3 Equipment-based objective-type epidural space detection*

1. Epidural waveform analysis
2. CompuFlo
3. Epidural stimulation test
4. Epidurography
5. Near-infrared tracking system
6. Epiduroscope

*3.3.4 Ultrasound-based objective-type epidural space detection*

1. Ultrasonography.

a. Preprocedural ultrasound scanning

b. Real-time ultrasound guidance

- Guidance positioning system for regional anesthesia (SonixGPS)
- Three- and four-dimensional real-time ultrasound
- Preprocedure 3D high-resolution images
- Machine vision
- Acoustic radiation force impulse (ARFI)

2. Doppler method.

## 4. Human-based subjective-type epidural space detection

### 4.1 Loss of air

It is the oldest and most common method followed for the loss of resistance technique to detect the epidural space [6]. This technique is done by filling air into syringe and connected to epidural needle to detect the loss of resistance.

Some complications are observed by the use of loss of resistance to air. They are pneumocephalus, air embolism, insufficient analgesia, delayed onset, higher incidence of dural puncture, nerve root compression, and subcutaneous emphysema [7].

### 4.2 Loss of fluid

Dogliotti described the loss of fluid technique in epidural space. He described that while advancing the needle by exerting the pressure on the piston of the syringe. Once this needle enters the epidural space, there is the sensation of needle slipping, simultaneous disappearance of resistance to injection, and the pressure felt on the piston of the syringe will disappear. He with his team also described about polyethylene catheter insertion to epidural space [8].

### 4.3 Saline with air bubble

Odom devised this method by attaching the capillary glass tube with air bubble and fluid. He modified the capillary method of saline with air bubble of 2 ml. He said that the movement of this air bubble to the needle indicates epidural space, and the movement of the air bubble away from the needle indicates subarachnoid space (dural tap) [9].

The fluid LOR does not provide the same feel as air for appreciating the LOR.

### 4.4 Lidocaine

2–3 ml test dose of lignocaine 1–2% confirms the epidural space. If the lidocaine is administered to subarachnoid space, there is be sudden onset of weakness in bilateral lower limbs, and it does not occur when it is administered into epidural space. This property is used as test dose to confirm the epidural space.

### 4.5 KSMM (The combined plunger pressure-manometer method)

It is a satisfactory alternative for the loss of resistance technique [10].

### 4.6 BiP test (Bidigital pressure test)

It is a simple procedure where pressures of two fingers are used to feel the LOR for epidural [11]. It is described that pressures of two fingers are adequate to feel the epidural space.

### 4.7 Use of hanging drop

Alberto Gutierrez discovered the hanging drop technique in February 1933. He was searching for epidural space with LOR technique with fluid. Due to stiff resistance, he removed LOR syringe and noted a small drop of liquid hanging at the tip of the needle. As he advanced the needle, the drop suddenly disappeared or moved inside the epidural space due to negative pressure of the epidural space [12].

### 4.8 CSF (Cerebral spinal fluid) ceased to drip

A method described by Sebrechts describes to do a dural tap in the beginning by inserting the needle into the subarachnoid space. Later, the needle is withdrawn until CSF ceased to drip to locate the epidural space [6].

### 4.9 Sterile water injection

Lund used 5 cc syringe filled with distilled water for epidural space identification. The distilled water causes burning pain if the patient is awake, and in asleep patient it causes slight movement [13]. It is due to irritation caused by sterile water in epidural space.

### 4.10 Loss of guidewire resistance (LOGR, epidural space finder)

The guidewire is used instead of air in the LOR technique. When the needle goes through the ligamentum flavum, there was constant rotation of dials on both sides leading to resistance of guidewire. Once the needle entered the epidural space, the dial lost the resistance and the guidewire moved a few centimeters into the epidural space [14].

### 4.11 Membrane in syringe technique

In this technique, a plastic membrane is placed in the middle of the syringe, dividing it into two compartments. The distal compartment of syringe has nozzle and is filled with saline. The proximal part of the syringe has plunger and is filled with air. Once this enters, the epidural space wrinkling of the plastic membrane is seen which can be appreciated by the loss of air. This technique also avoids injection of air into the epidural space. Even sometimes due to no appreciation of loss of resistance, the epidural space is identified by visible wrinkling of the membrane [15].

### 4.12 Epidural Queckenstedt test

Compression of bilateral internal jugular veins lead to increased subarachnoid pressures and increased epidural pressure which is used to confirm epidural puncture in this test [16].

### 4.13 Cold test

The injection of local anesthetic into epidural space gives a cold sensation in the back, and it is called as the cold test [17].

### 4.14 Hissing sound

In loss of resistance to air technique, once the needle enters the epidural space the air rushes into the epidural space. This is detectable on a stethoscope attached to epidural needle and audible as hissing sound [18].

### 4.15 Second needle method

After first needle LOR is obtained, the second needle LOR is obtained in the adjacent intervertebral space. If both these needles are in epidural space, 5 ml of rapid injection of normal saline from one needle will lead to fluid leakage from the other needle called the second needle method [19].

Current scientific evidence:

- False-positive LORs can happen in 17% of the patients. Saline with air bubble loss of resistance technique is preferred by most users.
- Studies are done to compare other syringes with epidural loss of resistance syringe, and it has been found to be 66–81% similar [20]. Hence, it is always better to use epidural loss of resistance syringe.
- Three different techniques were used for LOR assessment: incremental needle advancement with intermittent LOR assessment, continuous needle advancement with high-frequency intermittent LOR assessment, and continuous needle advancement with continuous LOR assessment. Postdural puncture headache is due to increased needle tip overshoot distance after LOR. Needle tip overshoot is defined as the distance traveled by the needle tip beyond the point where LOR can be first obtained. Of all the three techniques, incremental needle advancement with intermittent LOR assessment resulted in deepest needle tip overshoot [21]. The needle tip overshoot was less with continuous needle advancement with continuous loss of resistance assessment.
- Any drug or air pushed through the epidural space has a risk to enter the circulation and cause unwanted systemic effects. Hence, anesthesiologists should

be always cautious of the quantity of air pushed in epidural space and its placement [22].

Limitations and disadvantages of some popular techniques

There has been some explanation by MRI studies for false loss of resistance. Supraspinous ligament and interspinous ligament in lumbar region are biconcave axially. These gaps lead to deposition of anterior fat giving false loss of resistance [23].

The other causes of false-positive loss of resistance are as follows:

- Age-related cysts in interspinous ligaments seen in higher number of patients above 60 years;
- Paravertebral muscles give a false LOR;
- Frequent midline gaps hamper the gap between ligamentum flavum and epidural space;
- Intermuscular planes between the muscles.

## 5. Equipment-based subjective-type epidural space detection

These methods use equipments to detect the loss of resistance. It is not definitive that the loss of resistance is in epidural space. It is therefore highly subjective in the detection of epidural space.

### 5.1 Acoustic puncture assist device (APAD)

It documents pressure throughout the procedure of epidural. It provides real-time auditory and visual displays of pressure waveforms. It simultaneously uses three senses: hear (auditory signal), see (pressure and auditory graph on the screen), and touch (LOR from the needle) [24].

### 5.2 LOR technique with fluoroscopy

It is done in the prone position. Once the needle reaches L5-T1 interlaminar foramen, fluoroscopy of AP (anteroposterior) is done to confirm the placement. When LOR is done, lateral view of the fluoroscopy is done [25]. The disadvantage of this technique is patient needs to be put in prone position to undergo fluoroscopy.

### 5.3 EpiFaith syringe

The EpiFaith syringe has a spring-loaded plunger with the syringe. On the loss of resistance, the syringe moves by itself thus showing the epidural space [26].

### 5.4 Episure autodetect syringe

It is a spring-loaded loss of resistance syringe with a coaxial compression spring within a LOR syringe. This syringe gives constant pressure when it is being advanced.

Hence, the operator can use both his hands in advancing the needle [12]. To minimize the false loss of resistance, the episure syringe is attached to the needle once its tip is in the interspinous ligament as this does not detect epidural space, but it detects only the loss of resistance [27].

### 5.5 Epidrum

It contains a small drum with a diaphragm on one of its sides. The device is placed between Tuohy needle and syringe for epidural placement. On penetration of epidural space, there is sudden collapse of the diaphragm giving visual evidence confirming the loss of resistance. It takes less attempts and shorter time in comparison with standard LOR [28].

### 5.6 Epidural balloon

A small inflated balloon is attached to the hub of the epidural needle, while the epidural needle is being inserted. On obtaining the epidural space, the balloon collapses due to negative pressure [29]. A Y-shaped connector is attached to the epidural needle where the one end is having the balloon and the other end is attached to the syringe for charging the balloon. The balloon collapse on entering the epidural space is faster than traditional LOR giving a visual evidence of loss of resistance [30].

### 5.7 Electrocardiography (ECG)-guided system

In this system, the epidural tip is having or contains one of the ECG lead. Another surface electrode is positioned at desired dermatomal level. Once this ECG enabled epidural catheter reaches the desired segment, it matches with the reading of the surface electrode [31]. It confirms the needle entry into respective dermatomal level.

### 5.8 Drip infusion method

It combines method of LOR with drip infusion for confirmation of the epidural space. It identifies the true epidural space by LOR and later with fluid dripping present. In pseudo or false LOR, there is no fluid dripping [32].

Current scientific evidence:

- Less commonly used modern methods (epidrum, lidocaine, acoustic device, and Macintosh balloon) are better compared to air, saline, and both with relation to loss of resistance for the identification of epidural space [33].

- The risk of epidural vein cannulation is higher in sitting position (15.7%) in comparison with lateral position (3.7%) of the parturients. This study shows the correlation between posture and epidural catheter insertion [34]. Hence, in parturients, insertion of epidural needle insertion with catheter in lateral position is always preferred.

Limitations and disadvantages of some popular techniques

The advantage of ECG-guided epidural catheter is that it can be used in the presence of local anesthetic and neuromuscular blocking agents. This technique helps to match the vertebral level of particular dermatome but does not confirm its location in epidural space.

## 6. Equipment-based objective-type epidural space detection

These are the techniques or methods which take the help of equipments and identify the epidural space accurately most of the times.

### 6.1 Epidural waveform analysis

In the epidural pressure waveform, there is a drop in pressure once the catheter enters the epidural space. Epidural space pressure waveform and computed tomography cathetergram are helpful in identifying the epidural space and location of epidural catheters. It is obtained by transducing an epidural catheter. The pressure changes observed on epidural waveform when the needle went through ligamentum flavum is around 82 ± 25 mmHg. This pressure dropped to 6.5 ± 11.6 mmHg once the needle entered the epidural space [35]. The quantity of saline required for epidural waveform analysis is 5 ml.

The epidural pressure waveform analysis has reported 81% sensitivity, 100% specificity, 100% positive predictive value, and 17% negative predictive value [36].

### 6.2 CompuFlo

The CompuFlo epidural instrument is a computer controlled drug delivery system that can precisely measure the pressure of human tissues in real time at the tip of the needle. It gives real time exit-pressure data at the needle tip. Both visual and audio graphic of exit pressure is provided. With CompuFlo, the needle entry into the ligamentum flavum increase pressure and audible tone. Once it enters the epidural space there is a big drop in pressure and audiotone. A drop in pressure for more than 5 seconds confirms entry into epidural space [37, 38].

CompuFlo helps in identification of true loss of resistance by sudden and sustained drop (more than 5 seconds) in pressure (greater than 50% of maximum pressure) and pitch of audible tone with formation of low and stable plateau pressure. In case of false LOR any one of the above is not achieved. If the pressure increases after drop in pressure it is a false LOR [39].

### 6.3 Epidural stimulation test

It involves electrical stimulation of nerves passing through the epidural space. Motor or sensory response to stimulation of 1–10 mA indicates epidural location of catheter. Stimulation <1 mA happens when the catheter is in subarachnoid position, subdural space, or close to nerve root [40].

### 6.4 Epidurography

It is obtaining fluoroscopy of contrast dye administered through epidural catheter. Typical epidural spread can be appreciated on fluoroscopic image. Equipment required and radiation risks are the disadvantages of this technique [41].

### 6.5 Near-infrared tracking system

A fiberoptic wire is placed in an epidural catheter which emits infrared signal picked up by infrared camera. This infrared tracking system helps in the identification of the epidural space. In this technique, the signal is poor in obese patients, and when catheter passes under the lamina making it is difficult to track the epidural space [42].

### 6.6 Epiduroscope

It is a fiberscope or a camera which is advanced through the 18-guage Tuohy needle into the epidural space. The outer diameter of this scope is 0.8 mm [43]. This epiduroscope gives the visualization of the epidural space.

Current scientific evidence

Attempts were made to check the epidural pressure. It was found that at T3–T5 level, the median epidural pressure was 1 mmHg (−1 to 4.5 mmHg). The epidural pressure at T7–T10 level is 4 mmHg (2 to 7.8 mmHg). The subatmospheric epidural pressure is higher at mid-thoracic area in comparison with lower thoracic area [44]. The lumbar epidural pressure is greater than atmospheric pressure when referenced to zero at the dorsal spine level [45].

Limitations and disadvantages of some popular techniques

The CompuFlo can be used to localize the epidural space, but it does not decrease the overall catheter failure rate or accidental dural puncture rate. It does not help in the identification of midline or guide the trajectory of the epidural needle [46].

The epidural pressure waveform will not aid in the detection of subarachnoid, intravascular, or subdural catheter misplacement [47]. Hence, it is not cent percent effective in the confirmation of epidural space.

The disadvantages of epidural stimulation are that it becomes ineffective on the administration of local anesthetic, neuromuscular blocking agents, and in preexisting neuromuscular disease. It becomes ineffective in those conditions where the nervous system is affected.

## 7. Ultrasound-based objective-type epidural space detection

### 7.1 Ultrasonography

Two methods are used.

#### *7.1.1 Preprocedural ultrasound scanning*

A handheld ultrasound device for epidural identification—A wireless ultrasound device is used to limit the storage space for the ultrasound equipment. The software is programmed to calculate the depth of the epidural space. Horizontal and vertical lines are drawn from the midpoint to the probe at each inter spinous space. Later, the ultrasound device is kept aside. Using the marked lines, the epidural needle is inserted to the depth achieved by the ultrasound earlier to get the epidural space. The success of up to 87% has been achieved for the first pass of epidural needle to identify the epidural space by the ultrasound method [48].

#### *7.1.2 Real-time ultrasound guidance*

Though it is real-time placement of epidural catheter, two operators are considered necessary for real-time ultrasound guidance [49]. Some have reported that single person technique is possible by in-plane method, and it requires a lot of expertise in doing the same. There is also risk of ultrasound gel entering the epidural space [50].

Different types of ultrasound modalities are used to help localize the epidural space.

i. Guidance positioning system for regional anesthesia (SonixGPS).

   This uses an electromagnetic motion tracking system which helps in determining the position of the needle. It is more useful in out-of-plane approach [51].

ii. Three- and four-dimensional real-time ultrasound.

   Three- and four-dimensional real-time ultrasound has shown to help in regional anesthesia [52]. Certain difficulties are present in 3D/4D ultrasound images. They are varying bony shadows and artifacts due to complex anatomy of the spine. There are also problems with poor resolution, poor needle visibility, and reduced frame rate. Hence, it requires a high skill to perform the needle insertion into the epidural space.

iii. Preprocedure 3D high-resolution images.

   The preprocedure three-dimensionsl high-resolution images are constructed and later used in real-time 2D ultrasound image. This helps in the point of insertion of needle, trajectory of the needle, and depth of epidural space, making it more easier in getting the epidural space.

iv. Machine vision.

   The machine vision is a form of artificial intelligence where computer is helping to recognize images. It compares with previous stored data, and once familiar structures are recognized, they are pointed out by ultrasound image [53]. This artificial intelligence helps and gives clues to direct the epidural needle in the right direction and right depth. It helps by correlating the present ultrasound image with previous stored images.

v. Acoustic Radiation Force Impulse (ARFI).

   In the acoustic radiation force impulse (ARFI), the images are derived from differences in the mechanical properties of tissue rather than acoustic properties. It is used to know the tissue structural and mechanical properties.

In ARFI imaging plane, if imaging needles are out of required plane, the local stiffening effect of the needle can be visualized within ARFI imaging plane, thus helping in needle visualization [54].

### 7.2 Doppler method

The epidural needle is connected to a Doppler probe which is connected to a speaker and a paper recorder. On entry to epidural space through loss of resistance, "whoosh" sound is heard followed by spontaneous drop in Doppler flow tracing [55]. The appreciation of this sound helps in the identification of the epidural space.

Limitations and disadvantages of some popular techniques

The difficulty with real-time two-dimensional ultrasound is tracking of needle. From entry to epidural space is visualization of needle, or needle tip is difficult. This can be taken care with the help of needle tracking and navigation tools.

Needle visibility is a problem with ultrasound methods. Usually 2D B-mode ultrasound guidance is used for needle entry guidance to epidural space. The needle visibility is difficult when insertion angle is too steep, difference between imaging plane and needle plane and small needle gauge.

## 8. Future of epidural space detection

Raman spectroscopy has shown unique spectrum for all paravertebral and neuraxial tissue layers in porcine tissues [56]. Further studies of Raman spectroscopy is required on human subjects. If proved or invented, unique spectrum of Raman spectroscopy can be used to identify the epidural space.

Color flow Doppler function is being used to visualize the flow in epidural space on the injection of normal saline or air (1 ml over 1 second) [57]. Higher skills training is required, and it might require a long learning curve for expertise.

CompuFlo or technology built on the same with real ultrasound guidance could be the future instrument or technique of choice for difficult epidural.

Fiber Bragg grating (FBG) sensor for loss of resistance—This uses a novel soft system (SS) based on one fiber Bragg grating sensor (FBG) which is present in a soft polymeric matrix for LOR detection [58].

Ultrasound—Embedded needle is used for the identification of epidural space, and placement of catheter in real time with axial resolution of 0.15 mm has been tried on porcine models [59]. Further human trials are required to evaluate the effectiveness on humans.

Bioimpedance—Different tissues have different electrical impedance. This property helps to distinguish different types of tissues. Epidural space has higher fat content compared to nearby structures. This property could be utilized by bioimpedance in future to detect epidural space [60].

Optical spectroscopy—This method is tested on animal models. The needle is customized with optical fibers integrated into the cannula. The optical spectra (visible and near-infrared wavelength) are obtained at different depths. The estimates of blood and lipid volume fractions are determined. The lipid fractions obtained from epidural space were in the range of 1.9- to 20-fold higher than muscle, and epidural vein has high blood volume fraction [61].

Optical coherence tomography (OCT)—This is a type of B-mode ultrasonography using light reflection. This technology uses the light reflected to determine the depth of penetration to 2–7 mm to create the images of the tissue. This technology has helped to avoid neural damage in animal studies [62].

Due to reduced opportunities and to mitigate medical errors, simulation training for technical skills will help the trainees. To bridge the requirements and resources, multiple simulators from different manufactures are available in the market.

## 9. Conclusion

It has been more than 100 years since the discovery of LOR in epidural space, and we have not been able to find an ideal method to detect LOR space which has 100% specificity and 100% sensitivity and is safe and user-friendly. Research for better methods are still required to discover an ideal LOR instrument for the epidural space.

## Author details

Prashanth Jagadeesha Prabhu
Vydehi Institute of Medical Sciences and Research Centre, Bengaluru, India

*Address all correspondence to: prashanthjnpl@gmail.com

## References

[1] Hermanides J, Hollmann MW, Stevens MF, et al. Failed epidural: Causes and management. British Journal of Anaesthesia. 2012;**109**:144-154. DOI: 10.1093/bja/aes214

[2] Sicard JA, Forestier J. Radiographic method for exploration of the extradural space using Lipiodol. Revista de Neurologia. 1921;**28**:1264-1266

[3] Heldt TJ, Moloney JC. Negative pressure in epidural space: Preliminary studies. The American Journal of the Medical Sciences. 1928;**175**(3):371-376

[4] Tran DQH, Gonzalez AP, Bernucci F, et al. Confirmation of loss-of-resistance for epidural analgesia. Regional Anesthesia Pain Medicine. 2015; **40**:166-173. DOI: 10.1097/AAP.0000000000000217

[5] Elsharkawy H, Sonny A, Chin KJ. Localiation of epidural space: A review of available technologies. Journal of Anaesthesiology, Clinical Pharmacology. 2017;**33**(1):16-27. DOI: 10.4103/0970-9185.202184

[6] Durrans SF. High extradural segmental block. Anaesthesia. 1947;**2**(3): 106-111. DOI: 10.1111/j.1365-2044.1947.tb02082.x

[7] Figueredo E. Techniques for identifying the epidural space. Revista Española de Anestesiología y Reanimación. 2005;**52**(7):401-412

[8] Dogliotti AM, Ciocatto E. Method of differential block in pain relief. Anesthesiology. 1955;**16**:623-626. DOI: 10.1097/00000542-195507000-00018

[9] Odom CB. Epidural anesthesia. The American Journal of Surgery. 1936; **34**(3):547-558. DOI: 10.1016/S0002-9610(36)90679-7

[10] Bhate H. KSMM (kombinierte Stempeldruck- Manometer- Methode). [The combined plunger pressure-manometer method. A technique for identifying the peridural space]. Anaesthesist. 1992;**41**(4):224-227

[11] Carden E, Ori A. The BiP test: A modified loss of resistance technique for confirming epidural needle placement. Pain Physician. 2006;**9**(4):323-325

[12] Aldrete JA, Gutierrez VP. Alberto Gutierrez and the hanging drop. Regional Anesthesia and Pain Medicine. 2005;**30**(4):397-404. DOI: 10.1016/j.rapm.2005.04.006

[13] Lund PC, Cwik JC, Magaziner R. Epidural Anesthesia in general surgery. Anesthesiology. 1956;**17**:605-615. DOI: 10.1097/00000542-195607000-00012

[14] Yang J, Choi R, Cho K, et al. The development of a novel device based on loss of guidewire resistance to identify epidural space in a porcine model. Journal of Healthcare Engineering. 2020; **22**:8899628. DOI: 10.1155/2020/8899628

[15] Lin BC, Chen KB, Chang CS, et al. A 'membrane in syringe' technique that allows identification of the epidural space with saline while avoids injection of air into the epidural space. Acta Anaesthesiologica Sinica. 2002;**40**(2): 55-60

[16] Yokoyama T, Ushida T, Yamasaki F, et al. Epidural puncture can be confirmed by the Queckenstedt- test procedure in patients with cervical spinal canal stenosis. Acta

Anaesthesiologica Scandinavica. 2008; **52**(2):256-261. DOI: 10.1111/j.1399-6576. 2007.01506.x

[17] Sinha PK, Dubey PK. Prediction of successful epidural catheter placement by a "cold test". Anaesthesia and Intensive Care. 2006;**34**:31-35

[18] Mirakhur RK, Bandopadhyay A. Correspondence: An auditory guide to the location of the epidural space. Anaesthesia. 1973;**28**:707

[19] Davidson JT. Identification of the epidural space. Anesthesiology. 1966;**27**: 859

[20] Gladwin J, Maese S, Ballisat B. Investigating the use of non-loss of resistance syringes for epidural insertion: Experience on a mannequin. International Journal of Obstetric Anesthesia. 2022;**52**:103595. DOI: 10.1016/j.ijoa.2022.103595

[21] Cometa MA, Lope BM, Vasilopoulos T, et al. Does the technique for assessing loss of resistance Alter the magnitude of epidural needle tip overshoot? Simulation in Healthcare. 2020;**15**(3):154-159. DOI: 10.1097/ SIH.0000000000000419

[22] Jaffe RA, Siegel LC, Schnittger I, et al. Epidural air injection assessed by transesophageal echocardiography. Regional Anesthesia. 1995;**20**(2):152-155

[23] Lawrence S, Llewellyn S, Hunt H, et al. Anatomy of the lumbar interspinous ligament: Findings relevant to epidural insertion using loss of resistance. Regional Anesthesia and Pain Medicine. 2021;**46**(12):1085-1090. DOI: 10.1136/rapm-2021-103014

[24] Lechner TJ, van Wijk MG, Maas AJ. Clinical results with a new acoustic device to identify the epidural space. Anaesthesia. 2002;**57**:768-772. DOI: 10.1046/j.1365-2044.2002.02621.x

[25] Arici T. An operator's experience of the loss-of-resistance technique in epidural injections: An observational study. Eurasian Journal of Medicine. 2021;**53**(1):48-52. DOI: 10.5152/ eurasianjmed.2021.20014

[26] Athar MW, Guo N, Ortner C, et al. An observational pilot study of a novel loss of resistance syringe for locating the epidural space. International Journal of Obstetric Anesthesia. 2021;**47**:102984. DOI: 10.1016/j.ijoa.2021.102984

[27] Habib AS, George RB, Allen TK, et al. A pilot study to compare the Episure Autodetect syringe with the glass syringe for identification of the epidural space in Parturients. Anesthesia & Analgesia. 2008;**106**(2):541-543. DOI: 10.1213/ane.0b013e3181606c0a

[28] Sawada A, Kii N, Yoshikawa Y, et al. Epidrum: A new device to identify the epidural space with an epidural Tuohy needle. Journal of Anesthesia. 2012;**26**: 292-295. DOI: 10.1007/s00540-011-1278-1

[29] Macintosh RR. New inventions. Anaesthesia. 1950;**5**:97-99

[30] Fyneface-Ogan S, Mato CN. A clinical experience with epidural balloon in the localization of the epidural space in laboring parturients. Nigerian Quarterly Journal of Hospital Medicine. 2008;**18**:166-169. DOI: 10.4314/nqjhm. v18i3.45021

[31] Tsui BC, Seal R, Koller J. Thoracic epidural catheter placement via the caudal approach in infants by using electrocardiographic guidance. Anesthesia and Analgesia. 2002;**95**(2): 326-330. DOI: 10.1097/00000539-200208000-00016

[32] Ok SY, Ryoo SH, Baek YH, et al. Drip infusion method as a useful indicator for identification of the epidural space. Korean Journal of Anesthesiology. 2009; **57**(2):181-184. DOI: 10.4097/kjae.2009.57.2.181

[33] Carvalho LP, Agarwal A, Kashiwagi FT, et al. Commonly- used versus less commonly- used methods in the loss of resistance technique for identification of the epidural space: A systematic review and meta- analysis of randomized controlled trials. Journal of Clinical Anesthesia. 2017;**38**:41-51. DOI: 10.1016/j.jclinane.2017.01.017

[34] Harney D, Moran CA, Whitty R, et al. Influence of posture on the incidence of vein cannulation during epidural catheter placement. European Journal of Anaesthesiology. 2005;**22**(2): 103-106. DOI: 10.1017/s0265021505000190

[35] Gong Y, Shi H, Wu J, et al. Pressure waveform-guided epidural catheter placement in comparison to the loss- of-resistance conventional method. Journal of Clinical Anesthesia. 2014;**26**(5): 395-401. DOI: 10.1016/j.jclinane.2014.01.015

[36] de Medicis E, Pelletier J, Martin R, et al. Technical report: Optimal quantity of saline for epidural pressure waveform analysis. Canadian Journal of Anaesthesia. 2007;**54**(10):818-821. DOI: 10.1007/BF03021709

[37] Capogna G, Coccoluto A, Capogna E, et al. Objective evaluation of a new epidural simulator by the CompuFlo epidural instrument. Anesthesiology Research and Practice. 2018;**2018**: 4710263. DOI: 10.1155/2018/4710263

[38] Capogna G, Camorcia M, Coccoluto A, et al. Experimental validation of the CompuFloA epidural controlled system to identify the epidural space and its clinical use in difficult obstetric cases. International Journal of Obstetric Anesthesia. 2018;**36**: 28-33. DOI: 10.1016/j.ijoa.2018.04.008

[39] Vaira P, Camorcia M, Palladino T, et al. Differentiating false loss of resistance from true loss of resistance while performing the epidural block with the CompuFlo epidural instrument. Anesthesiology Research and Practice. 2019;**2019**:5185901. DOI: 10.1155/2019/5185901

[40] Tsui BC, Gupta S, Finucane B. Confirmation of epidural catheter placement using nerve stimulation. Canadian Journal of Anaesthesia. 1998; **45**:640-644. DOI: 10.1007/BF03012093

[41] Uchino T, Hagiwara S, Iwasaka H, et al. Use of imaging agent to determine postoperative indwelling epidural catheter position. Korean Journal of Pain. 2010;**23**:247-253. DOI: 10.3344/kjp.2010.23.4.247

[42] Chiu SC, Bristow SJ, Gofeld M. Near-infrared tracking system for epidural catheter placement: A feasibility study. Regional Anesthesia and Pain Medicine. 2012;**37**:354-356. DOI: 10.1097/AAP.0b013e31824c0310

[43] Imai M, Kemmotsu O. Direct observation of the epidural space by the superfine fiberscope. Masui. 1992;**41**: 474-479

[44] Visser WA, Gielen MJM, Giele JLP, et al. A comparison of epidural pressures and incidence of true subatmospheric epidural pressure between the mid-thoracic and low-thoracic epidural space. Anesthesia and Analgesia. 2006;**3**(5): 1318-1321

[45] Thomas PS, Gerson JI, Strong G. Analysis of human epidural pressures. Regional Anesthesia. 1992;**17**(4):212-215

[46] Fiol AG, Aymen A. Identification of the epidural space with all the bells and whistles. International Journal of Obstetric Anesthesia. 2018;**36**:131-132. DOI: 10.1016/j.ijoa.2018.08.006

[47] Ghia JN, Arora SK, Castilo M, et al. Confirmation of location of epidural catheters by epidural pressure waveform and computed tomography cathetergram. Regional Anesthesia and Pain Medicine. 2001;**26**:337-341

[48] Seligman KM, Weiniger CF, Carvalho B. The accuracy of a handheld ultrasound device for Neuraxial depth and landmark assessment: A prospective cohort trial. Anesthesia and Analgesia. 2018;**126**(6):1995-1998. DOI: 10.1213/ANE.000000000 0002407

[49] Grau T, Leipold RW, Fatehi S, et al. Real-time ultrasonic observation of combined spinal-epidural anaesthesia. European Journal of Anaesthesiology. 2004;**21**:25-31. DOI: 10.1017/ s026502150400105x

[50] Tran D, Kamani AA, Al-Attas E, et al. Single-operator real-time ultrasound-guidance to aim and insert a lumbar epidural needle. Canadian Journal of Anaesthesia. 2010;**57**: 313-321. DOI: 10.1007/s12630-009-9252-1

[51] Wong SW, Niazi AU, Chin KJ, et al. Real-time ultrasound-guided spinal anesthesia using the SonixGPS needle tracking system: A case report. Canadian Journal of Anaesthesia. 2013;**60**:50-53. DOI: 10.1007/s12630-012-9809-2

[52] Belavy D, Ruitenberg MJ, Brijball RB. Feasibility study of real-time three–/four-dimensional ultrasound for epidural catheter insertion. British Journal of Anaesthesia. 2011;**107**: 438-445. DOI: 10.1093/bja/aer157

[53] Tran D, Rohling RN. Automatic detection of lumbar anatomy in ultrasound images of human subjects. IEEE Transactions on Biomedical Engineering. 2010;**57**(9):2248-2256. DOI: 10.1109/TBME.2010.2048709

[54] Rotemberg V, Palmeri M, Rosenweig S, et al. Acoustic radiation force impulse (ARFI) imaging- based needle visualization. Ultrasonic Imaging. 2011;**33**:1-16. DOI: 10.1177/ 016173461103300101

[55] Nader-Djalal N, Reddy R, Bacon DR. Doppler guidance for epidural catheter placement. Regional Anesthesia and Pain Medicine. 1998;**23**:326-328

[56] Anderson A, Kang JW, Gubin T, et al. Raman spectroscopy differentiates each tissue from the skin to the spinal cord: A novel method for epidural needle placement? Anesthesiology. 2016;**125**(4): 793-804

[57] Bosch OFC, Gleicher Y, Arzola C, et al. Color flow Doppler in spinal ultrasound: A novel technique for assessment of catheter position in labor epidurals. Regional Anesthesia and Pain Medicine. 2022;**47**(12):775-779. DOI: 10.1136/rapm-2022-103948

[58] Tommasi FD, Presti DL, Virgili F, et al. Soft system based on Fiber Bragg grating sensor for loss of resistance detection during epidural procedures: In Silico and In vivo assessment. Sensors (Basel). 2021;**21**(16):5329. DOI: 10.3390/ s21165329

[59] Chiang HK, Zhou Q, Mandell MS, et al. Eyes in the needle: Novel epidural needle with embedded high-frequecy ultrasound transducer—Epidural access in porcine model. Anesthesiology. 2011; **114**:1320-1324. DOI: 10.1097/ ALN.0b013e31821b5746

[60] Kalvoy H, Frich L, Grimnes S, et al. Impedance-based tissue discrimination for needle guidance. Physiological Measurement. 2009;**30**(2):129-140. DOI: 10.1088/0967-3334/30/2/002

[61] Rathmell JP, Desjardins AE, van der Voort M, et al. Identification of the epidural space with optical spectroscopy: An in vivo swine study. Anesthesiology. 2010;**113**:1406-1418. DOI: 10.1097/ALN.0b013e3181fcee47

[62] Raphael DT, Yang C, Tresser N, et al. Images of spinal nerves and adjacent structures with optical coherence tomography: Preliminary animal studies. The Journal of Pain. 2007;**8**:767-773. DOI: 10.1016/j.jpain.2007.04.006

Section 2

# Pharmacology of Epidural Medications

Chapter 3

# Physiology and Pharmacology of Epidurally Administered Drugs

*Katarina Tomulić Brusich, Lara Valenčić and Željka Polonijo*

## Abstract

In the last few decades, epidural administration of various drugs has gained popularity and widespread clinical acceptance. Epidural administration of local anesthetics and opioids has been considered "state of the art" in acute pain management (thoracic and major abdominal surgery, labor). Its advantage is that it yields profound, long-lasting, dose-dependent analgesia, leaving other sensory and motor functions intact. It facilitates early patient mobilization and ambulation and therefore reduces the risk of postoperative thromboembolism and respiratory complications. The increment in the elderly population caused an increase in musculoskeletal and spine diseases and thus, epidural steroid injections have become highly effective for chronic pain treatment. There are many factors that have an impact on drug physiology and pharmacology in the epidural space and, therefore, can modify epidural anesthesia or the expected effect of another medication. This chapter provides insight into this complex and comprehensive topic to demonstrate a predictable pattern that can provide a safe and accurate guide to clinical practice.

**Keywords:** epidural space, pharmacology, opioids, local anesthetics, steroids

## 1. Introduction

Clinical indications for epidural anesthesia and analgesia have expanded over the years. Epidural analgesia is often used as a supplement to general anesthesia for surgical procedures in pediatric and adult patients [1, 2]. It is well tolerated in patients with age-related comorbidities, such as chronic obstructive pulmonary disease, hypertension, coronary artery disease, and renal insufficiency [3, 4]. Elderly patients may benefit from decreased postoperative confusion and delirium associated with regional anesthesia if intraoperative hypotension is avoided [5].

Epidural drug administration provides analgesia in intraoperative, postoperative, peripartum, and end-of-life settings. It can be used as the primary anesthetic for surgery from the mediastinum to the lower limbs. Additionally, epidural techniques are increasingly being used for diagnostic procedures, acute pain therapy, and the management of chronic pain [6]. Epidural anesthesia reduces surgical stress response, the risk of cancer recurrence, the incidence of perioperative thromboembolic events, and, possibly, the morbidity and mortality associated with major surgery [7–9].

Aforesaid is in the ideal setting. However, epidural drug administration and its clinical effect may face many obstacles compared with subarachnoid block, since epidural space is "virtual" and somewhat different from spinal space. Injection of the drug in a large volume is made into the region where target nerves are entrenched behind barricades and where blood flow inflicts heavy losses on the advancing local anesthetic. Furthermore, the flow of fluids in the epidural space is modified by abdominal and thoracic pressures transmitted through the intervertebral lamina. All mentioned can affect and modify drug pharmacology and clinical effect.

One of the first articles written on epidural drug physiology and pharmacology was by legendary professor Bromage, who set the cornerstone of regional anesthesia [10]. Since then, the principle has remained the same. However, new drugs were reinstated, and many randomized studies have been undertaken for a better understanding of this complex subject.

This chapter provides insight into this complex and comprehensive topic in order to demonstrate a predictable pattern that can provide a safe and accurate guide to clinical practice.

## 2. "Back to basics"

### 2.1 Anatomy of epidural space

Before pharmacology issues are discussed, it is important to regard the site of administration and relevant anatomy in some detail. The vertebral column has 7 cervical, 12 thoracic, 5 lumbar, 5 fused sacral, and most commonly, 4 fused coccygeal vertebrae. Vertebral anatomy varies according to each level. The atlas (C1) and the axis (C2) are highly atypical vertebrae, but from C3 downward the vertebrae have a recognizable anterior body, posterolateral pedicles, transverse processes, and posterior laminae, which fuse to form the spinous processes. The spinal canal enclosed within these structures is known as the epidural space. Its central portion is occupied by the dural sac, which contains the anterior and posterior spinal nerve roots, also known as the caudal equina. Between the arachnoid and the pia mater, which is applied to the spinal cord, is cerebrospinal fluid (**Figure 1**) [11].

The epidural space surrounds the dura mater circumferentially and extends from the foramen magnum to the sacrococcygeal ligament. Posteriorly it is bound by the ligament flavum, laterally by the pedicles and the intervertebral foramina, and anteriorly by the posterior longitudinal ligament, respectively [1].

Each intervertebral foramen connects the epidural with the paravertebral space without any barrier. Even within the intervertebral foramen, the epidural space is perforated by a spinal nerve and its duplicated dura sheath. Furthermore, the epidural space is in connection with the paravertebral space and attached anatomical structures. Thus, the epidural space is neither a distinct anatomical compartment nor a homogeneous compartment [12]. Disk herniation (the most common chronic disease of the spine) occurs primarily at weak points in this posterior longitudinal ligament in an area that comprises the anterior epidural space, as opposed to the more clinically relevant posterior epidural space [12].

The epidural space contains adipose tissue, blood vessels, nerve roots, lymphatics, and various haphazard fibrous connections to the ligament flavum, which can have an unpredictable effect on the course of an epidural catheter. The ligament flavum is not uniform from skull to sacrum, nor even within an intervertebral space. The ligament thickness, distance to the dura, and skin-to-dura distance vary with the area of the vertebral canal (1.5–3.0 mm in cervical, 3.0–5.0 mm in thoracic, 5.0–6.0 mm in

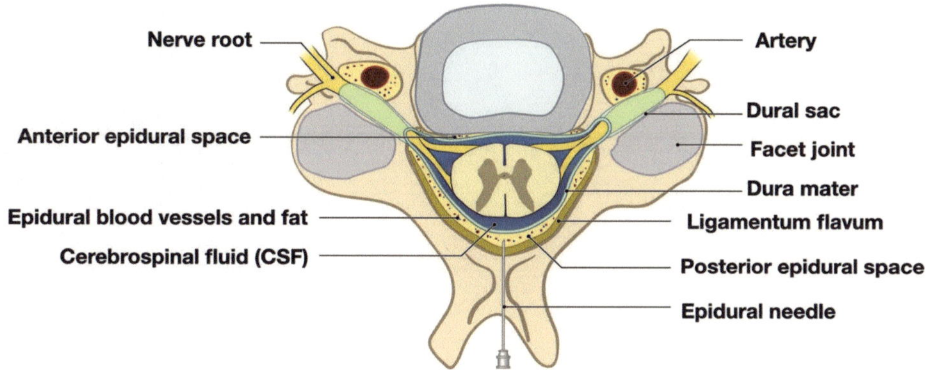


**Figure 1.**
*Anatomy of the spinal cord (cross-sectional view). Notice the close proximity of the posterior epidural space to the subarachnoid space.*

lumbar, and 2.0–6.0 mm in caudal level, respectively) [13]. The amount of adipose tissue in the epidural space appears to affect the spread of local anesthetic, but it remains unclear whether epidural fat prolongs nerve block duration by serving as a reservoir or decreases the amount of available drug, thereby slowing onset or both. The reduction of adipose tissue with age is speculated to account in part for the higher levels and faster onset of epidural anesthesia in the elderly [14]. Also, those fat pads under the ligament flavum could further explain the inhomogeneous spread of a local anesthetic and the deviation of epidural catheters. They can influence catheter advancement and may facilitate catheter migration through the intervertebral foramen [15].

Epidural arterial supply arises from anterior and posterior spinal arterial arcades, arising from spinal arteries entering the space through every intervertebral foramen. Its venous drainage is *via* a plexus of valveless veins, which is in the anterior epidural space. The venous plexus receives blood shunted from thoracic and pelvic veins, which means that straining and coughing can transiently engorge them. Because the plexus is valveless, blood from any of the connected systems can flow into the epidural vessels. Therefore, in situations when caval flow is obstructed, as in late pregnancy, the spinal veins are distended and occupy an abnormal absorption of the spinal canal [11, 12].

Aforesaid, the epidural space is irregular and segmental. It is distensible and an injection of fluid tends to distort its dimensions. Rheumatoid arthritis and trauma may affect this relationship and the ability to recognize the relevant anatomy [16]. We think that a picture tells a thousand words (**Figure 2**). With this kind of spine pathology, the epidural administration will probably modify or alter the detection of epidural space, epidural catheter placement, and drug efficacy. Also, we can expect a high incidence of epidural insertion-related complications [11, 12, 15].

## 2.2 Physiologic effects of epidural blockade

The extent of these physiologic effects depends on the level of placement and the number of spinal segments blocked. In general, high thoracic epidural nerve blocks (i.e., above Th5) and extensive epidural nerve blocks are associated with more profound physiologic changes than nerve blocks with low sensory levels (i.e., below Th10). Spinal anesthesia and epidural anesthesia produce a similar degree of differential sensory blockade. Epidural anesthesia produces a sympathetic block, which

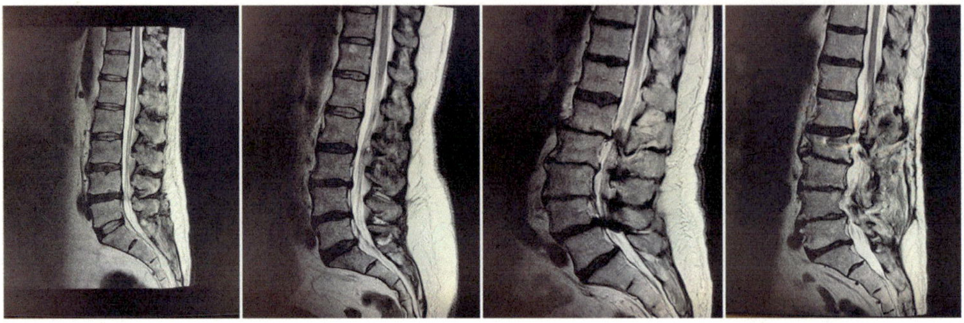

**Figure 2.**
*MRI of the lumbar spine (T2-weighted sagittal) shows mild to severe lumbar pathology (from left to right). Courtesy of Department of Radiology, Clinical Hospital Centre Rijeka.*

extends higher than the sensory block, with the lack of motor block, which is characteristic of spinal anesthesia [17].

The nerve fibers vary in their response to LAs based on their diameter and state of myelination. The most susceptible are Aδ nociceptive fibers (which are responsible for autonomic nervous system transmission) resulting in an epidural block in a concentration-dependent manner [18]. The meaning of the aforementioned is that this type of myelinated fiber requires larger LA concentrations because of the myelin sheath, also becomes blocked faster, and recovers faster. On the other hand, small unmyelinated C-fibers (postganglionic fibers in the autonomic nervous system and nerve fibers at the dorsal roots) that are in charge of transmission of visceral dull pain sensation need lower concentrations of LAs because they lack a protective myelin sheath and diffusion barrier, but with the longer necessary time to recover. Based on these findings, differential neural block and sensitivity to LAs are best presented in an epidural block where the main goal is to achieve appropriate anesthesia in a dermatomal distribution of the patient's pain complaints [19]. We can say succinctly that in the epidural block, autonomic fibers (types C and B) are the fastest and easiest blocked nerve fibers, and usually reach higher dermatome levels (2–6 levels) than the sensory block. Myelinated, Aδ nociceptive fibers are the next fibers where the neuronal transmission stops; sensory functions include first temperature (cold), then the pain (pinprick), and finally, touch. The last ones blocked are the proprioception (A-beta, Aβ) and motor fibers (Aα) with a descending dermatomal level [18, 20].

During general anesthesia combined with epidural analgesia, the degree of sedation and minimum alveolar concentration (MAC) sparing effect appear to correlate with the height and level of the sensory nerve block. Also, a thoracic block is associated with a greater sedative effect than the lumbar block and a higher concentration of LAs may contribute to a greater MAC-sparing effect. The addition of opioid adjuvants to the epidural LA solution does not appear to reduce volatile agent requirements any further, although it does contribute to better postoperative pain scores [21].

Cardiovascular and hemodynamic effects are primarily the result of a sympathetic nerve fiber blockade. They include venous and arterial vasodilation, reduced systemic vascular resistance, and changes in chronotropy and inotropy resulting in blood pressure and cardiac output variations. The type and intensity of these changes are related to the level of nerve block, the total number of dermatomes blocked, as well as the type and dose of LA administered. In general, high thoracic nerve blocks can cause marked changes compared with lumbar blocks [22].

Epidural anesthesia may also affect lung function, depending on the level of block. Tidal volume remains unchanged, while vital capacity and forced expiratory volume in 1 s (FEV (1.0)) can be decreased during high thoracic epidural block [23]. However, thoracic epidural anesthesia has benefits in major abdominal and thoracic surgery since it enhances pain relief postoperatively and thus reduces postoperative pulmonary complications [24].

As for the gastrointestinal (GI) system, sympathectomy associated with an epidural block in the mid-to-low thoracic levels results in unopposed vagal tone, which manifests clinically with increased peristalsis, relaxed sphincters, an increase in GI secretions, and, likely, more rapid restoration of GI motility in the postoperative phase [25].

Because renal blood flow is maintained through autoregulation, epidural anesthesia has little effect on renal function in healthy individuals. Compensatory and feedback mechanisms (afferent arteriolar dilation and efferent arteriolar vasoconstriction) ensure constant renal blood flow over a broad range of pressures (50–150 mmHg) [26].

As far as thermoregulation is concerned, hypothermia is primarily due to peripheral vasodilation resulting in heat redistribution from the core to the periphery. In addition, reduced heat production (due to reduced metabolic activity) results in a negative heat balance [25].

Epidural anesthesia reduces the hypercoagulable state in the postoperative period and is associated with a decreased risk of deep vein thrombosis (DVT) and pulmonary embolism. Likewise, it could effectively inhibit central sensitization and reduce the damage of intraoperative stress response to cognitive function [27].

### 2.3 Basic epidural pharmacology

When drugs are administered neuraxial, it is of crucial importance to understand the pharmacokinetics and pharmacodynamics of the agents employed in order to ensure adequate anesthesia/analgesia as well as safety. In general, neuraxial administered drugs need to reach their primary site of action to work [28]. Absorption to the main target site (i.e., the spinal cord and intrathecal dorsal nerve root as well as local and systemic (re-)distribution) determine the onset and duration of action of epidural and intrathecal drugs.

After injection of epidural drug(s), the drug solution coats the dural sack, spreading up and down in a fairly random fashion. From the epidural space, drugs may go four ways (**Figure 3**):

1. Exit the intervertebral foramina to reach the paraspinous muscle space

2. Distribute into epidural fat. This defines the main influence on epidural drug behavior. The drug forms a reservoir and redistributes gradually, creating a longer effect. The speed of onset is also mainly related to lipid solubility (discussed later in the chapter).

3. Diffuse into ligaments

4. Diffuse across the spinal meninges and into the cerebrospinal fluid (CSF) where the arachnoid is the main meningeal barrier to diffusion. Apart from that, a small minority of drugs will penetrate the systemic circulation and then appear in the CSF after diffusing out of the spinal cord.

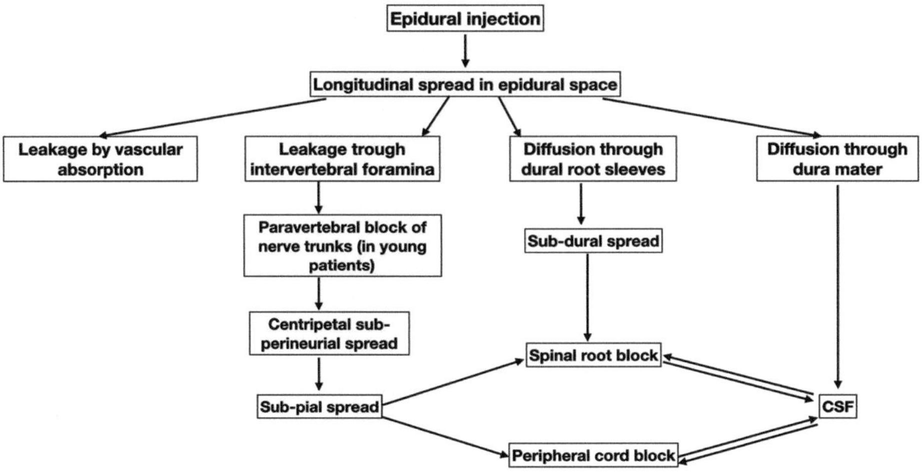


**Figure 3.**
*The fate of an epidural injection; CSF—Cerebrospinal fluid [10].*

In the epidural space, diffusion has the main influence on drug absorption and is done according to Fickian principles. The main factors that influence the penetration of an epidurally administered drug into the cerebrospinal fluid (CSF) are as follows:

**Dose, volume, and concentration**: The dose of LAs necessary for epidural anesthesia or analgesia is a function of the concentration of the solution and the volume injected. The concentration of the drug affects the density of the nerve block; the higher the concentration, the more profound the motor and sensory nerve block. Volume and total LA dose are the variables that affect the degree of spread of the nerve block. A larger volume of the same concentration of LA will block a greater number of nerve segments. However, if the total dose of LA is unchanged, but the concentration is doubled, the volume can be halved to achieve a similar spread of LA. Clinical observations of the spread of epidural analgesia have shown that the extent of the segmental blockade is mainly determined by the mass of the drug injected (the product of volume and concentration) and not by volume alone. Another interesting finding regarding epidural space is that, beyond a certain point, further increase in anesthetic concentration does not consistently reduce the time required for anesthesia to develop, nor produce an improvement in the rather merger quality of motor blockade [29]. These findings reveal an unexpectedly complex relationship between concentration and effect and support the suggestion that epidural blockade is not a simple matter of diffusion from one space to another, but rather of several diffusion pathways (**Figure 3**).

**Surface area** is largely determined by the volume of the infused drug.

**Protein binding** determines the free fraction of the drug.

**Lipid solubility** is defined by the ionization constant (pKa value) of the drug and the pH of the solution.

General guidelines for the administration of epidural drugs state that 1–2 mL of medications should be applied per segment until the target dermatomal level is reached. In the group of patients of lower height, a reduction to 1 mL per segment is recommended [30]. The established term "time to two-segment regression" is defined as the time required for the regression of the sensory block at two dermatomal levels, and it varies depending on the type of applied LA in the epidural block. It requires the repeated application of one-half or one-third of the given initial dose [31].

### *2.3.1 Epidural pharmacology of local anesthetics (LAs)*

For local anesthetics (LAs), the most relevant properties are the ionization constant (pKa value), lipophilicity, and the degree of protein binding. LAs are defined as water-soluble salts of lipid-soluble alkaloids. Their structure consists of three components: a lipophilic aromatic ring, an intermediate ester or amide chain, and a terminal hydrophilic amine group. All mentioned components contribute to distinct properties of the molecule [32]. The aromatic ring as a lipophilic structure improves the liposolubility of the molecule. This characteristic allows diffusion through the myelin sheath and also correlates with potency because a greater dose of LA can enter the neuronal fiber [32, 33].

The intermediary chain categorizes LAs into esters or amides with their characteristics (**Table 1**) [33].

While the potency of LAs is related to its lipid solubility (those with higher lipid solubility more easily permeate neuronal membranes), the speed of onset predominantly depends on the pKa (a lower pKa would effectuate a higher speed of onset), and the duration of action is significantly influenced by the degree of protein binding, more precisely on alpha-1-glycoprotein (increased protein binding is associated with a longer duration of action and lower bioavailability [18, 34]). The LA base is stable in a solution as a hydrochloride salt (a weak base). At the time of injection, LAs are in the ionized, quaternary, water-soluble state and not able to diffuse through the myelin sheath. So, the time of onset of anesthesia is directly related to the proportion of molecules that convert from quaternary to the tertiary, lipid-soluble, non-ionized structure when they are exposed to the physiologic pH of 7.4.

That is determined using the ionization constant (pKa) for the LAs, and it is presented and calculated using the Henderson-Hasselbach equation for weak bases [18, 32, 33]:

$$\log\left(\frac{non-ionized}{ionized} form\right) = pKa - pH \tag{1}$$

At normal and physiological pH of 7.4, 50% of LAs exist in a tertiary, lipid-soluble non-ionized form, and 50% are in the quaternary, a water-soluble ionized form; only 50% of molecules can diffuse through both the epineurium and the neuronal membrane. When the pKa of the LA is close to the physiological pH, the onset of action is the fastest due to the optimal ratio of non-ionized and ionized fractions. Acidosis in the surrounding tissue (such as infection) increases the ionized fraction of the LAs, making them water-soluble with no diffusion capacity through the myelin sheath. Once the molecule reaches the tertiary form in the axoplasm of the neuron, the amine gains a hydrogen ion and, now ionized and in a quaternary form again, it is responsible for the actual blockade of the VGSC. So, in conclusion, the equilibrium between quaternary and tertiary forms lies in the pH of the tissues and the pKa of the anesthetics [33]. An optimal anesthetic uptake and activity require a relatively low pH at the site of action [35].

### *2.3.2 Epidural pharmacology of opioids*

Concerning opioids, lipid solubility is the essential determining factor for pharmacological effects after neuraxial application. Generally speaking, opioids

| Classification | pKa | Relative potency* | Onset | Duration (min) | Maximum single dose (mg) | Epidural administration |
|---|---|---|---|---|---|---|
| ESTERS | | | | | | |
| Procaine | 8.9 | 1 | Slow | 45–60 | 500 | No |
| 2-Chloroprocaine | 8.7 | 2 | Rapid | 30–45 | 600 | Yes |
| Tetracaine | 8.5 | 8 | Slow | 60–180 | 100 (only topical) | No |
| AMIDES | | | | | | |
| Lidocaine | 7.9 | 2 | Rapid | 60–120 | 300 | Yes |
| Etidocaine | 7.7 | 2 | Slow | 240–480 | 300 | Yes |
| Prilocaine | 7.9 | 2 | Slow | 60–120 | 400 | Yes |
| Mepivacaine | 7.6 | 2 | Slow | 90–180 | 300 | Yes |
| Bupivacaine | 8.1 | 8 | Slow | 240–480 | 175 | Yes |
| Levobupivacaine | 8.1 | 8 | Slow | 240–480 | 175 | Yes |
| Ropivacaine | 8.1 | 6 | Slow | 240–480 | 200 | Yes |

**Relative potency varies based on the route of administration.*

**Table 1.**
*Classification of LAs with their main characteristics.*

are lipid-soluble weak bases that are highly bound to the proteins and are ionized at physiologic pH. The variations in protein binding affinity are the main reason for the different speeds of transfer across the cellular membrane [36, 37]. Hydrophilic opioids such as morphine have a slower onset and a longer duration of action, while lipophilic opioids such as fentanyl and sufentanil produce a rapid onset and shorter duration of action. Lipophilic opioids tend to accumulate in fat-rich tissues such as epidural fat and white matter of the spinal cord, resulting in smaller concentrations in cerebrospinal fluid (CSF). They have less bioavailability, a large volume of distribution, and a larger initial volume in the central compartment compared with more hydrophilic molecules such as morphine [38–41]. Neuraxial lipophilic opioids have a more rapid distribution and clearance from the spinal cord and epidural space than hydrophilic opioids, resulting in a lower rate of respiratory depression and sedation [42, 43].

Elimination of epidurally administered opioids varies related to the molecular weight of the drugs and is dependent on the speed at which opioids spread in the rostral direction. Their mechanism of action is dose-dependent. In small doses, they show spinal effects, whereas in higher doses, they are responsible for supraspinal analgesia and can have pronounced systemic side effects [38–40].

It appears that the systemic absorption of drugs from the epidural space follows a two-compartment model. The rapid disappearance phase is believed to be related to uptake by rapidly equilibrating tissues (i.e., tissues that have high vascular perfusion). The slower phase of disappearance is mainly the function of the particular compound and the half-life of the drug. LAs appear in the venous blood within a few minutes of epidural injection and rises to a maximum in 10–30 minutes, depending upon the diffusion characteristics of the drug concerned [44]. Lipophilic drugs are also readily cleared into the plasma and can hence produce undesired side effects in the central nervous system. The degree of absorption depends on the dose and the presence or absence of vasoconstriction in the epidural solution. Very large doses may cause sufficiently high blood levels to produce a toxic reaction [45].

### *2.3.3 Other factors that may affect epidural block onset*

**Height** is very poorly correlated with epidural dose requirements except for extremely tall or short patients [30, 46].

**Weight:** There is little correlation between the spread of analgesia and the weight of the patient. However, in morbidly obese patients, there may be compression of the epidural space related to increased intra-abdominal pressure and, therefore, a higher nerve block may be attained with a given dose of LA [46].

**Age:** With advancing age, the LA dose required to attain a specific nerve block is reduced. Greater spread in the elderly may be related to the reduced size of the intervertebral foramina, which theoretically limits the regress of LAs from the epidural space. Decreased epidural fat, which allows more of the drug to bathe the nerves, and changes in the compliance of the epidural space may lead to enhanced cranial spread and prolonged duration of the block [47]. This results in a possible need for up to 40% less volume of administrated epidural medications in elderly patients [48].

**Pregnancy:** Dose requirements at term are reduced by about one-third to one-half. Two reasons may be responsible: First, the pregnant uterus causes a partial occlusion of the inferior vena cava at term, and the proportion of the venous returns from the legs, and pelvis is diverted into the internal vertebral plexus. This results in the enlargement of the extradural veins and the reduction of the remaining volume in the epidural space [49]. Second, pregnancy causes increased sensitivity to both LAs and general anesthetics. The possible mechanism is attributed to elevated levels of progesterone and endogenous endorphins, which leads to increased permeability of membranes and blood vessels [50].

**Blood flow:** The natural factors that impair blood flow in the epidural space such as age, arteriosclerosis, and diabetes increase the spread of analgesia, but they do not carry with them the tendency for a more profound block. Additionally, arterial hypertension may prolong blockade, but its effects on the quality of blockade have not been sufficiently investigated [51].

**Epidural catheter positioning:** Epidural block height is affected primarily by the level of injection. In the cervical region, drugs administered in the epidural space mostly spread caudally, while in the midthoracic region (level of Th2–Th6), the expansion is equally cranial and caudal. By administering the epidural drugs in the lower thoracic region (Th6-L1), the spread is only cranial. After a lumbar epidural, the spread is more cranial than caudal with a delay in the onset of anesthesia at the L5-S1 segments because of the larger size of these nerve roots. The position of the patient on the bed does not affect the spread of the medications in the epidural space, regardless of whether the patient is in a sitting or lateral position [30, 31, 48].

In summary, the onset of epidural blockade is relatively slow, due to the fact that administered drugs have to pass several diffusion barriers. The result depends upon interaction of many different factors discussed above. The epidural blockade is indeed a complex process, which takes place at many different sites, including spinal roots, nerve trunks, and the spinal cord itself. There are still many gaps in our knowledge of the fundamental process of epidural action, which requires further investigations, careful experimental design, and examination of direct and indirect evidence from clinical and laboratory sources due to the fact that many variables are not susceptible to direct measurement. It is very difficult to meet all the specified criteria, and much of the proposed research did not acquire ethical committee approval. This is probably the reason why the majority of the literature on basic epidural pharmacology is of an older date.

## 3. Epidural administration of local anesthetics

Epidural anesthesia has gained great importance due to its safety, especially when using local (LAs) anesthetics in combination with opioids that have become commonplace for relief of pain. Synthetic opioids can, thereby, increase the effectiveness of anesthetics, leading to the main goal of epidural medication administration, which is the patient's maximum pain relief [52].

### 3.1 Nerve anatomy and physiology

The main role of LAs is to inhibit action potential in nociceptive fibers and block the transmission of pain impulses. The abovementioned effect is achieved by suppressing action potentials in excitable tissues by blocking voltage-gated sodium ($Na+$) channels (VGSC) [18].

Surgical incision creates trauma to the affected tissue, activating in that way nociceptors, leading to, in the literature, the so-called "inflammatory soup." Nociceptors are the free endings of one form of myelinated A fibers called A-delta ($A\delta$) fibers that can be found in the skin, muscles, joints, bones, and viscera. Every stimulation of nociceptors (like surgical incision) results in depolarization with activation of Na + channels—a structure that is composed of a large pore-forming alpha ($\alpha$) subunit associated with one or two beta ($\beta$) subunits. The $\alpha$ subunit has four domains (I–IV), each containing six segments (S1–S6). The segments S5 and S6 form the channel, such as the short loops of amino acids that link them. The voltage-sensitive region is S4 in each domain containing positively charged arginine or lysine amino acids. Looped domains III and IV are meritorious for gate inactivation (**Figure 4**) [18].

Normally, these channels can exist in three states: resting, open, and inactivated. During the rest, entry of Na + ions is denied, and the channel is in a non-conductive state. This makes a membrane potential of approximately −70 mV. Stimulation of the channel, the great influx of Na + ions occurs, and the S4 segments open by outward spiral rotation, initiating depolarization. Following the sudden change in membrane voltage, the Na + channel assumes an inactivated state. The Na + channel inactivation and efflux of potassium ($K+$) ions restore the electrochemical gradients and depolarize the nerve back to its resting state [18, 53].

### 3.2 Selection of LAs

The epidural anesthesia is produced by the diffusion of LAs through the dura mater achieving their effects on nerve roots and in paravertebral space passing through the intervertebral foramina [32]. Commonly used LAs for an epidural block can be divided into short-, intermediate-, and long-acting (**Table 1**). The time required to achieve peak performance varies on the type, dose, and volume of LA, which is administered into the epidural space. The time to onset of epidural block after injection of LAs can usually be detected within 5–10 minutes [20, 32].

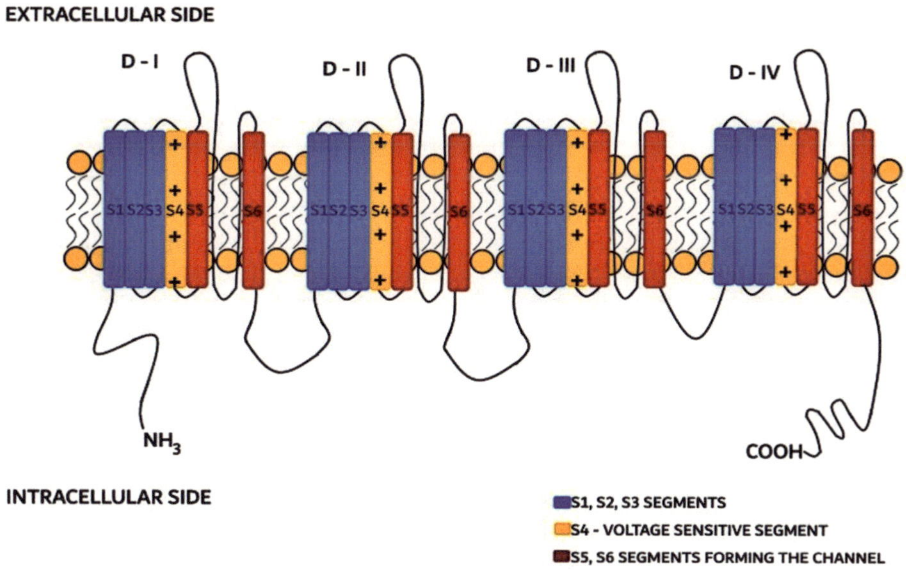


**Figure 4.**
*Structure of voltage-gated sodium (Na+) channel (VGSC) with main subunits and segments.* **Legend:** *Blue—S1, S2, S3 segments, yellow—voltage-sensitive segment S4, red—S5,6 segments forming the channel.*

The most common application of short-acting ester LA, 2-chloroprocaine is neuraxial anesthesia because of its short duration. The United States Food and Drug Administration (FDA) recently approved 2-chloroprocaine for providing neuraxial anesthesia for adults undergoing short-duration abdominal and lower extremity surgery. Throughout the world, 2-chloroprocaine is used off-label when the fast onset of epidural anesthesia is indicated, like in obstetric settings, for the need for an emergency cesarean section, but it is pregnancy category C. Its high pKa of 8.7 is an exception to the abovementioned rule of faster onset of LAs when they are closer to physiological pH. The 2-chloroprocaine has a very low risk for systemic toxicity because it is rapidly hydrolyzed by pseudocholinesterase, so it can be administrated in higher doses and have a faster onset, regardless of pKa [54].

Lidocaine is the intermediate-acting LA that is used commonly for surgical anesthesia *via* the epidural route. It is classified as an amide LA agent and also a class Ib antiarrhythmic agent on the Vaughan-Williams classification. Usually, it is combined with epinephrine, so the duration of action can be extended up to 60%. Lidocaine has a pKa of 7.7, meaning that approximately 25% of molecules will be able to diffuse through the myelin sheath, so it has a more rapid onset of action than other LAs with higher pKa (except 2-chloroprocaine). For the epidural block, it is usually used in a 1–2% concentration in a plain form or, more often, with a 1 per 200,000 epinephrine [55].

Long-acting LAs used for epidural blocks are bupivacaine, levobupivacaine, and ropivacaine. Because of the long duration of action, for many years, bupivacaine has been used as the first LA of choice for an epidural block. Today, the doses of this amide LA used for an epidural block are associated with a higher risk for cardiac toxicity because of its interaction with cardiac Na + channels, such as central nervous system (CNS) toxicity with an unwanted postoperative motor blockade. Due to the aforementioned and the need for a smaller dose and volume, bupivacaine is the ideal choice for spinal anesthesia [32, 56]. It has a higher pKa than other local anesthetics and consequently a slower onset of anesthesia. It can be prepared in three different concentrations: 0.25%, 0.5%, and 0.75%. A concentration of 0.5% is the most suitable for surgical anesthesia and epidural block. Accidentally injected intravenously, 0.75% bupivacaine has been associated with refractory cardiac arrest, and it is no longer recommended for epidural block [48]. Levobupivacaine, the S (−)-enantiomer and racemic sibling of bupivacaine, has similar characteristics as bupivacaine but with less pronounced cardiotoxic effects. Equal doses of levobupivacaine and bupivacaine can provide similar onset and duration of anesthesia (up to 6–8 hours) but with fewer life-threatening side effects and a better safety profile with levobupivacaine [57]. Likewise, levobupivacaine and ropivacaine also present a long-acting, amide LA that is enantiomerically pure (S-enantiomer) with properties and efficacy similar to bupivacaine. Because of its low lipid solubility, ropivacaine has a lower potency than bupivacaine but with a higher affinity for Aδ and C fibers than those controlling motor functions like Aβ, so it can easily produce the earlier mentioned differential block. Ropivacaine is less cardiotoxic than equal concentrations of racemic bupivacaine, and it has a significantly higher threshold for CNS toxicity [58, 59]. Ropivacaine offers an advantage concerning cardiotoxicity when applied and compared with bupivacaine, but with a marginal advantage in a differential block and with a higher market price. The duration of anesthesia for all long-acting anesthetics is between 6 and 8 hours [48].

In conclusion, levobupivacaine is imposed as the safest and most suitable long-acting LA for use in the epidural block.

### 3.3 Adverse effects of local anesthetics

Improper handling of LAs can lead to both systemic and local toxic effects [18].

#### *3.3.1 Local anesthetic systemic toxicity (LAST)*

This life-threatening event is most often the result of the intravascular application of LA (e.g., unintentional epidural vein cannulation during catheter placement) or in less common situations as a result of excessive concentration after LA absorption at the injection site. The extent of this effect depends on the dose of the LA, the site of application, and the fact whether a vasoconstrictor such as epinephrin was included in the solution. The most common consequences are visible in the CNS and cardiovascular system. High plasma concentrations of LAs lead to the blockade of cortical inhibitory pathways by interrupting neuronal depolarization. In the clinical picture, the abovementioned are manifested in the early phase as dizziness, tinnitus, perioral paresthesia and tingling, audio-visual disturbances, agitation, and confusion of patient. As concentrations get higher, generalized seizures appear with the further possibility of a state of consciousness disturbances, coma, and respiratory arrest. Simultaneously, in the cardiovascular system, rhythm disturbances are the most likely disorders as a consequence of a direct blockade of myocardial Na + channels leading to prolonged PR, QRS, and ST intervals. That can manifest as re-entry tachy- and bradyarrhythmias with hypotension, and eventually, cardiac arrest, which most often results in asystole [31, 60, 61].

When long-acting anesthetics are desired, it is better to use levobupivacaine or ropivacaine because of their higher threshold for CNS and cardiovascular complications, such as lower vasodilatory properties and slower systemic absorption. Maximal

| | Epidural | Intrathecal |
|---|---|---|
| Absorption into target site | Rate of diffusion into CSF is slower, and depends on Fick principles:<br>- Volume (surface area of available meninges)<br>- Concentration<br>- Lipophilicity (pH, pKa)<br>- Protein binding and free fraction<br>- CSF flow rate/turbulence | Rate of diffusion into target tissue is rapid:<br>High CSF concentration<br>Short diffusion distance (2–4 mm) |
| Local distribution | Epidural spaces are irregular, segmental, and the injected material encircles the dural sack | Depends on basicity (density of inject ate relative to CSF) |
| Systemic distribution | Two competent model: rapid early distribution (into epidural fat) and then slowly back out | Slow absorption; increased half life<br>The more lipophilic the drug, the faster it is cleared from the CSF |
| Metabolism and elimination | Normal mechanism prevails (liver and kidney). However, because of the hemodynamic effect of spinal (anesthetic) drugs, the perfusion of liver and kidneys may be decreased, which could delay clearance. | |

**Table 2.**
*Epidural vs. intrathecal drug administration [30].*

single doses of each local anesthetic must be respected (**Table 2**). This condition must be treated timely, including airway maintenance, suppression of seizure activity, and hemodynamic support with preparation for possible cardiopulmonary resuscitation [61]. Lipid emulsion (20%) therapy should be started according to the American Society of Regional Anesthesia (ASRA) guidelines, as follows:

For a patient over 70 kilograms—a rapid 100 mL bolus of emulsion over 2–3 minutes followed by another 200–250 mL over 15–20 minutes [19].

For patients below 70 kilograms—an initial loading dose of 1.5 mL/kg over 2–3 minutes, followed by a continuous infusion of 0.25 mL/kg/min for a minimum of 10 minutes after restoring circulatory stability [19].

The recommended dosing limit is 12 mL/kg for repeated bolus doses [62].

### *3.3.2 Local tissue toxicity*

All LAs possess nerve and muscle toxicity that can be, in a rare number of cases, clinically apparent. As the dose of LA gets higher, so as the duration of exposure, some local reactions such as nerve ischemia and nerve vulnerability are possible, and must be recognized promptly [48].

## 4. Epidural administration of opioids

One of the main priorities in current anesthesia practice is perioperative pain management, due to the fact that inadequately treated pain is associated with increased morbidity, mortality, protracted recovery, and delayed discharge from the hospital. The main group of medications used for the treatment of acute and chronic pain is opioids, which achieves their effect by binding to opioid receptors [36, 37, 63]. Opioids can be endogenous (i.e., enkephalins, endorphins, and endomorphins dynorphins) and exogenous (morphine, heroin, meperidine, fentanyl, and many others). Endogenous opioids are peptides that are expressed in pain pathways and packaged in core vesicles and transported to axon terminals during which they are broken down into smaller, more specific peptides, which eventually bind to the opioid receptors [37]. Exogenous opioids are derived from the opium poppy plant, more specifically alkaloid morphine, which can be processed to produce heroin and other synthetic opioids, and codeine and thebaine, which are used to produce drugs such as oxycodone, hydrocodone, and hydromorphone. The basic opioid molecule is morphine and most of the opioids that are used today in anesthesiology share its structural features and are made by complex alterations of the morphine molecule [36, 37, 63].

### 4.1 Opioid receptors

Opioid receptors, which are responsible for the main pharmacological effect of opioids, are a G-protein-coupled family of receptors. They have seven transmembrane portions; intra- and extracellular loops, extracellular N terminus, and intracellular C terminus. Opioid agonists bind to the receptor and activate the three subunits of the G-protein. The effects produced are mostly inhibitory, and they lead to the hyperpolarization of the cell and reduction of its excitability (**Figure 5**) [36, 37, 63, 64].

Four main types of opioid receptors have been identified—mu (μ), kappa (κ), delta (δ) opioid receptors (mu—MOR, kappa—KOR, and delta—DOR), and nociceptin (NOR) receptors. Other types of receptors that are proposed to exist are epsilon (ε) receptor, zeta (ζ) receptor, and a binding site called lambda (λ). Sigma (σ) receptors are not considered opioid receptors anymore but target sites for phencyclidine (PCP) and are responsible for psychomimetic effects, dysphoria, and depression (**Table 3**) [36, 37, 63, 64].

Opioid receptors are localized in and outside of the central nervous system (CNS). In the CNS, they are mainly located in the dorsal horn of the spinal cord and the cerebral cortex, thalamus, area postrema, the limbic system and the periaqueductal gray region, locus ceruleus, rostral ventral medulla, and peripheral afferent nerves. Outside of the CNS, they can be found in many other tissues such as the

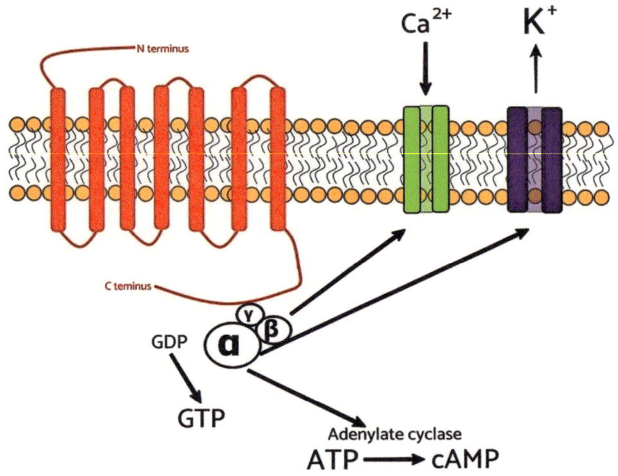


**Figure 5.**
*Structure of opioid receptor: Seven transmembrane portions, intra- and extracellular loops, extracellular N terminus, and intracellular C terminus. Opioid agonists bind to the receptor and activate three subunits of the G-protein. Production of cAMP decreases by inhibition of adenylyl cyclase, Ca2+ influx decreases by the closing of voltage-sensitive calcium channels, and K+ efflux increases.*

| Opioid receptor | Prototype agonist | Location | Effects |
|---|---|---|---|
| *Mu (μ) receptors (MOR)* | Morphine | Central nervous system<br>Cerebral cortex<br>Amygdala<br>Periaqueductal gray<br>Basal ganglia | Supraspinal analgesia<br>Euphoria<br>Sedation<br>↓Respiration<br>↓Gastrointestinal movements<br>Physical addiction<br>Miosis<br>Pruritus<br>Anorexia<br>Vasodilatation |
| *Kappa (κ) receptors (KOR)* | Ketocyclazocine | Diencephalic areas<br>Limbic areas<br>Spinal cord Brain stem | Spinal analgesia<br>Sedation<br>Dysphoria<br>Dependence<br>Dyspnea<br>↓Respiration |
| *Delta (δ) receptors (DOR)* | Delta-alanine-delta-leucine-enkephalin | Brain | Analgesia<br>↓Gastrointestinal movements |
| *Nociceptin receptors (NOR)* | Nociceptin/orphanin | Central nervous system | Analgesia<br>Hyperalgesia |

**Table 3.**
*Types of opioid receptors [36, 37, 63–65].*

gastrointestinal or biliary, and some of the actions of the agonists of these receptors outside of the CNS account for the adverse effects of opioids [36, 37, 63, 64].

Opioids are classified by their actions on opioid receptors as agonists, mixed agonists-antagonists, partial agonists, and antagonists [36, 37, 63].

Opioid agonists in the spinal cord inhibit the release of substance P from sensory neurons of the dorsal horn, changing the transfer of painful stimuli to the brain. In the brain stem, they modulate nociceptive transfer in the dorsal horn through descending inhibitory pathways. They change the response to pain in the forebrain and also induce activity in reward structures in the brain. Therefore, opioids provide analgesia by attenuation of peripheral nociceptive stimuli and by changing our central response to it. Agonists of MOR receptors mostly treat pain sensations carried by unmyelinated C fibers. Other sensations such as touch and temperature are not affected. With larger doses administered, they also produce drowsiness and sleep, but they do not affect responsiveness and amnesia. Through cough centers in the medulla, they produce antitussic effects, but also can sometimes produce a paradoxical increase in coughing after usage as an intravenous induction agent [36, 37, 63–65].

### 4.2 Adverse effects and metabolism of opioids

One of the most frequent and significant adverse effects of opioids is depression of ventilation. Opioids alter the ventilatory response to carbon dioxide in arterial blood, and they depress the hypoxic drive to breathing and diminish the ventilation drive in the patient. This effect is greater in patients who receive high dosages of opioids, are older, use other central nervous system depressants, and have renal or hepatic insufficiency [36, 37, 63–66].

Also, opioids produce vasodilatation by decreasing the central vasomotor tone in the brainstem and by directly acting on the blood vessels. They affect both preload and afterload. In older, hypertensive patients or patients with congestive heart failure, opioids can lead to significant hypotension [36, 37, 63, 64].

One of the most often associated adverse effects of opioid administration is nausea and vomiting, by stimulating the trigger zone in the area postrema in the fourth ventricle of the brain and pruritus, by weakening inhibition of itching by neurons of the dorsal horn in the medulla. These effects are the result of the rostral spread of opioids, meaning that more hydrophilic opioids tend to have these adverse effects when administered epidurally [36, 37, 41, 63–65].

Opioids affect the gastrointestinal system in a way that they cause tonic contractions of smooth muscles and decrease peristaltic, which can lead to the postoperative development of ileus. They can also lead to urinary retention by decrease in bladder detrusor tone and increase in urinary sphincter tone. This can be more pronounced in male patients when opioids are given epidurally or inthrathecally [36, 37, 41, 63–66].

The use of opioids in obstetric patients may affect neonates. It may inhibit or enhance the progress of labor. Also, possible is neonatal morbidity because of vascular reabsorption of drugs and possible transfer to the placenta and the fetus, which can lead to respiratory depression in neonates, neurological depression, and other side effects [66].

Opioids can produce alterations in body temperature, most likely by interacting with opioid receptors in the spinal cord and possibly by migration of the drug into the hypothalamus. Administration of epidural sufentanil decreases shivering and may induce hypothermia [66].

Opioids may also lead to different types of cardiac dysrhythmias and may lead to damage to the spinal cord (motor and sensory dysfunction), most likely due to the effect of opioid preservatives or additives, which leads to vasoconstriction and spinal cord ischemia [66].

All of these side effects are mediated *via* opioid receptors, and their treatment are opioid receptor antagonists such as naloxone. Administration of a pure antagonist may lead to the end of analgetic effects, and if this effect should be maintained, an opioid agonist/antagonist can be administered. Antiemetics are useful in treating nausea and vomiting, such as transdermal scopolamine patches in those receiving epidural morphine or droperidol in the epidural infusion [66, 67].

### 4.3 Types of opioids and elected representatives

By their origin, opioids are classified as follows:

1. Naturally occurring opioids:

    a. benzylisoquinolines (papaverine)

    b. phenanthrenes (morphine, codeine, oxycodone, hydrocodone)

2. Semi-synthetics: morphine derivatives with simple or complex changes

3. Synthetic opioids:

a. morphinan derivatives (i.e., levorphanol)

b. diphenyl or methadone derivatives (i.e., methadone)

c. benzomorphans (i.e., pentazocine, phenazocine)

d. phenylpiperidine derivatives (meperidine, fentanyl, sufentanil, remifentanil, alfentanil)

Tramadol is an atypical opioid, a partial agonist that also has central GABA, serotonergic, and catecholamine activity [36, 37, 63, 64].

#### *4.3.1 Morphine*

Morphine is considered a prototype opioid substance against which all others are evaluated (**Figure 6**). It consists of a benzene ring with two hydroxyl groups (a phenolic at the third position and an alcohol at the sixth position and the nitrogen atom). Both of these can be converted to ethers or esters. Many of the opioids that are used today in anesthesiology share their structural features, and also many of the semi-synthetic ones are created by modifications of morphine molecule [36, 37, 43–45].

It has a very slow onset time, is almost completely ionized at physiologic pH, has very low lipid solubility and high protein binding, and is rapidly conjugated with glucuronic acid. Therefore, it has a prolonged latency to peak effect, and it slowly penetrates the CNS. The non-alkalized form of morphine crosses the blood-brain barrier much easily. When given intrathecally or epidurally, it also has a slower onset and longer duration of action compared with more lipophilic opioids [36, 37, 43–45, 63, 64].

Its slow onset can lead to the stacking of doses in patients with severe pain. Since morphine is a high histamine releaser, it can cause hypotension, bronchospasm, and direct respiratory depression. Decreased sympathetic nervous system tone can lead to other already described side effects such as nausea, vomiting, pruritus, constipation, and miosis [36, 37, 43–45, 63, 64].

#### *4.3.2 Methadone*

Methadone is considered the best treatment option for opioid addicts since it has long-acting pharmacokinetics and a very rare development of withdrawal syndrome. It also acts as an NMDA receptor antagonist resulting in attenuated opioid tolerance and can be used in the treatment of severe neuropathic and opioid-resistant pain due to serotonin and norepinephrine reuptake inhibition. It has high lipid solubility (analgesic action 4–8 hours) and a very long elimination phase with a long half-life (up to 150 hours). It is considered to be a good analgesic alternative for patients with morphine allergies since it is unrelated to standard opioids in structure. It can be used epidurally with relatively fewer side effects than morphine. However, its use is still considered off-label [36, 37, 43, 45, 63, 64, 68, 69].

#### *4.3.3 Fentanyl*

Fentanyl can be administered in multiple ways; intravenously, through the skin, mucous membranes, lungs, and nasally, and also intrathecally and epidurally. It is

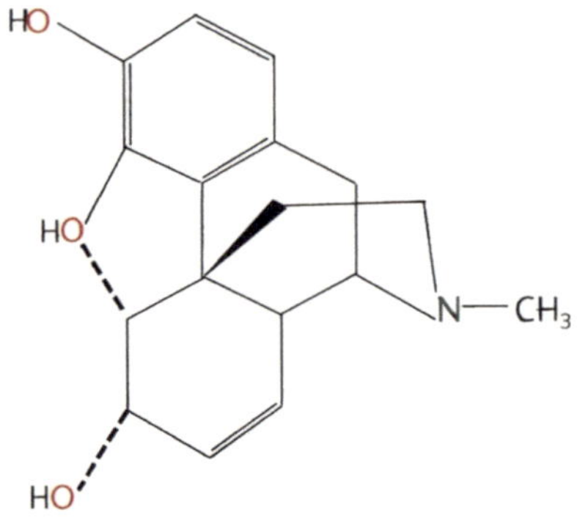


**Figure 6.**
*Structure of the morphine molecule: A benzene ring with two hydroxyl groups (a phenolic at the third position and an alcohol at the sixth position and the nitrogen atom).*

the oldest synthetic piperidine agonist and much more potent than morphine (80 times). It is highly lipophilic and binds strongly to proteins in the plasma (around 80%). The first-pass effect is mostly mediated by the lungs. It is primarily a MOR opioid agonist, and through this effect, it increases the pain threshold. Its duration of action is related to redistribution in highly vascular structures. It is metabolized in the liver and excreted *via* the kidneys, and it can be detected in urine 48 hours after administration [36, 37, 45, 63, 64, 70].

### *4.3.4 Alfentanil*

Alfentanil has a short terminal half-life after an intravenous bolus injection because it has a high diffusibility fraction and quickly reaches peak effect concentrations. It is lipophilic and has one-fourth or one-tenth the potency of fentanyl. A very high proportion of the drug is uncharged at physiologic pH. The effects of alfentanil are mediated through mu-opioid receptors, but cause more significant respiratory depression than fentanyl [36, 37, 45, 63, 64].

### *4.3.5 Sufentanil*

Sufentanil is the most potent opioid used in modern anesthesia (5–10 times more potent than fentanyl). It has a smaller volume of distribution and a terminal half-life between fentanyl and alfentanil. Like other fentanyl analogues, it is lipophilic. It has minimal cardiovascular side effects, preserving cardiac output and oxygen balance of the myocardium. It causes much harsher respiratory depression and rigidity of muscles compared with fentanyl [36, 37, 45, 63, 64, 70, 71].

### *4.3.6 Remifentanil*

Remifentanil is the shortest acting synthetic opioid available because it is very quickly hydrolyzed by tissue and plasma esterases. It has a short latency to peak effect and has a rapid effect. It is twice more potent as fentanyl and 100–200 times more potent than morphine. It does not accumulate in the tissues, and its duration of action does not increase with the duration of administration [36, 37, 45, 63, 64, 70].

#### *4.3.7 Hydromorphone*

Hydromorphone has been used epidurally in thoracic, abdominal, and pelvic surgery, post-Cesarean section, and post-laminectomy syndrome. It is a lipophilic agent that has a faster onset of analgesia than morphine and a longer duration of action than fentanyl. Also, it has fewer side effects than morphine [44, 72].

#### *4.3.8 Oxycodone*

Oxycodone has high bioavailability, faster analgesia onset, and less histamine release than morphine, but a much shorter duration of action. It has liposolubility similar to morphine. Some studies show that epidural administration of oxycodone has better analgetic outcomes than oxycodone given intravenously. However, its epidural administration has not been approved by the FDA [42, 45, 73, 74].

#### *4.3.9 Naloxone*

Naloxone is an opioid antagonist that binds to opioid receptors competitively, and it can reverse all effects of opioids if there is ongoing opioid therapy. Mostly, it is used to reverse opioid-induced ventilator depression. It is rapidly metabolized in the liver, has a high clearance, and mostly has a significantly shorter action than that opioid whose effect it has to reverse [36, 37, 63, 64].

#### *4.3.10 Nalbuphine, buprenorphine, pentazocine, and butorphanol*

Nalbuphine, buprenorphine, pentazocine, and butorphanol are partial agonist-antagonists that bind to opioid receptors. Buprenorphine is a kappa receptor antagonist and mu receptor agonist, while others listed are kappa receptor partial agonists and competitive mu antagonists. They are efficient in relieving mild and moderate pain and have less effect on ventilatory depression in patients (**Table 4**) [36, 37, 63, 64].

When different opioids are selected, one has to keep in mind how quickly the desired effect should be achieved, how long it must continue for, should the desired effect be quickly modified, and is there a need to completely avoid the adverse effects. Also, the route of administration is very important to achieve a steady state and achieve the desired effects.

## 5. Epidural steroid injection (ESI)

Corticosteroids are very attractive as drugs for many musculoskeletal diseases because of their potent anti-inflammatory effect. Epidural steroid injection (ESI) is widely used to treat various back pain conditions such as herniated intervertebral disc and spinal stenosis [75].

Initially, it was thought that the radicular pain was due to a compression of the nerve secondary to degenerative disc disease. However, recent studies show that inflammation plays a major role in the evolution of radiculopathy [76]. Clinically, a large herniation of an intervertebral disc associated with significant neural compression may be asymptomatic, whereas severe radicular pain may exist without

| Opioid type | pKa | Unionized at 7,4 pH (%) | Plasma protein bound (%) | Octanol/ water partition coefficient | Receptor affinity | FDA approved for epidural |
|---|---|---|---|---|---|---|
| Morphine | 8,0 | 23 | 20–40 | 1,4 | μ +++<br>κ +<br>δ | Yes |
| Methadone | 9,2 | 1 | 85–90 | 117 | μ +++<br>κ<br>δ | No |
| Fentanyl | 8,4 | 9 | 84 | 813 | μ +++<br>κ<br>δ | No |
| Alfentanil | 6,5 | 90 | 92 | 145 | μ +++<br>κ<br>δ | NA |
| Sufentanil | 8,0 | 20 | 93 | 1778 | μ +++<br>κ +<br>δ + | Yes |
| Remifentanil | 7,1 | 68 | 80 | 17,9 | μ +++<br>κ<br>δ | NA |
| Hydromorphone | 8,2 | | 20 | 1,3 | μ +++<br>κ<br>δ | No |
| Oxycodone | 8,5 | | 45 | 0,7 | μ ++<br>κ<br>δ | NA |

**Table 4.**
*Opioid physicochemical and pharmacokinetic properties. The octanol/water partition coefficient is a measure between the lipophilicity and hydrophilicity of a substance (value >1 = substance more soluble in fat-like solvents; < 1 = more soluble in water [36, 42–47].*

detectable root compression. Also, the size or shape of herniation and its eventual change do not correlate with clinical presentation or course [77]. The leak of the nucleus pulpous of the disc causes the release of several neuropeptides such as substance P, vasoactive intestinal peptide, calcitonin gene-related peptide and also nitric oxide, tumor necrosis factor α, metalloproteinases, and the production of hyperalgesic prostaglandins, thromboxanes, and leukotrienes. These cytokines activate immune cells and cause the attraction of lymphocytes, macrophages, and fibroblasts, leading to ischemia and inflammation. These biological components sensitize free nerve endings and adjacent nerve roots or dorsal root ganglions, producing back pain [78].

Corticosteroids belong to the class of steroid hormones produced by the cortex of the adrenal gland and are involved in several physiological regulatory mechanisms. They achieve the effect by the abolition of the rate-limiting step by the enzyme phospholipase A2 (PLA2) to liberate arachidonic acid from cell membranes. Arachidonic acid then leads to the upregulation of the cyclooxygenase and lipoxygenase enzymes, achieving the physiological effect by reducing intraneural edema, venous congestion, ischemia, and pain through the production of hyperalgesic prostaglandins, thromboxanes, and leukotrienes [78]. They are classified into glucocorticoids and mineralocorticoids. Glucocorticoids participate in the metabolism of carbohydrates, fats, and proteins with their anti-inflammatory action as is mentioned above. In epidural injection, glucocorticoids are routinely used and treated as epidural steroids. Current evidence suggests that more soluble glucocorticoids have a shorter duration of systemic effect than less soluble glucocorticoids [79]. On the other hand, mineralocorticoids play a role in the regulation of water and electrolytes in the body. In **Table 5**, physiochemical properties of corticosteroids are displayed.

Patients suffering from back pain with a radicular component due to herniated nucleus pulposus benefit the most from epidural steroid injection (ESI). The contraindications for ESI include local infection, systemic infection, allergy to injectate, and potentially bleeding disorders or anticoagulation. Contraindications for steroid injections can also expand to certain medical conditions, such as poorly controlled diabetes, hypertension, or congestive heart failure [80].

ESI utilizes the principle of delivering steroids directly to the source of the problem to create higher local concentrations. There are three most common routes for epidural steroid administration: the caudal route, the interlaminar approach, and the transforaminal approach [81]. Each of these routes has benefits, risks, and concerns regarding the efficacy of ESI. The caudal and interlaminar approach can lead to wide fluctuations in results due to an inability to deliver medication to the target area, and the drug spread can be affected by the presence or absence of epidural ligaments and scarring (post-surgical). In transforaminal injections, flow is set toward the anterior and lateral epidural space, while in the caudal and interlaminar route, flow is predominantly into the posterior epidural space and, therefore, away from probable sites of inflammation. Post-surgical patients cause problems due to loss of normal anatomy, landmarks, scarring, and poor flow within the space. Therefore, fluoroscopic-guided procedures enhance safety and improve the accuracy of placing the steroid at or nearer the site of the pathology [82].

Common ESI complications include hypothalamic-pituitary-adrenal (HPA) axis suppression, adrenal insufficiency, iatrogenic Cushing's syndrome, hyperglycemia, osteoporosis, and immunological or infectious diseases. The type of corticosteroid also affects the severity of complications. It is reported that HPA axis suppression was more likely with longer-acting insoluble corticosteroid formulations such as methylprednisolone or triamcinolone than betamethasone and dexamethasone [79]. The HPA axis suppression is observed in all patients who receive ESI and serves as an indicator of an ESI limitation. The recovery curve of HPA function after ESI is similar to that of the elimination of epidurally injected steroids and represents a dose-response relationship, which provides important information about the minimal dosage of epidural steroids [83]. However, the incidence of complications related to epidural steroids is not high, and most of them are not serious.

Risks associated with the needle placement or with injectate include infection (more common in immunocompromised patients and can include epidural abscess and meningitis) and bleeding (epidural hematoma occurs in ~0.02% of procedures). Several cases of spinal cord ischemia after ESI have been reported since they were first described [84]. The current hypothesis is that this is due to a particulate steroid suspension being injected into a small artery, which then causes the development of an anterior spinal artery syndrome.

The corticosteroids for ESI are divided into **particulate** (triamcinolone and methylprednisolone) and **non-particulate** (dexamethasone and betamethasone) formulations. There have been no serious complications attributed to the use of

| Name | Glucocorticoid potency (anti-inflammatory potency) | Mineralocorticoid potency (Na + retaining potency) | Duration of action (t1/2) (h) | Equivalent dose (mg) | Particulate or non-particulate | Particle size (mcg) |
|---|---|---|---|---|---|---|
| Hydrocortisone (cortisol) | 1 | 1 | 8 | 20 | P | Not studied |
| Prednisolone | 4 | 0.8 | 16–36 | 5 | P | Not studied |
| Methylprednisolone | 5–7.5 | 0.5 | 18–40 | 4 | P | <7.6 |
| Triamcinolone | 5 | 0 | 12–36 | 4 | P | 0.5–100 |
| Dexamethasone | 25–80 | 0 | 36–54 | 0.75 | Non-P | <7.6 |
| Betamethasone | 25–30 | 0 | 36–54 | 0.75 | P | 0.5–100 |

**Table 5.**
*Physicochemical properties of corticosteroids [85].*

non-particulate steroids (dexamethasone). There is evidence that only dexamethasone and methylprednisolone have particles consistently smaller than a red blood cell (7.5–7.8 μm) but that methylprednisolone tended to aggregate and pack densely with a possible propensity to cause emboli and block a small arteriole, whereas dexamethasone did not (**Table 5**). It is also important to note that dexamethasone is a water-soluble preparation, whereas methylprednisolone is a suspension. Therefore, dexamethasone is generally considered safer as it is water-soluble and does not aggregate and pack densely and, for practical purposes, is considered non-particulate in the field of chronic pain management [85]. Recent literature documents that there is no significant difference in pain relief at any point between non-particulate and particulate steroids. There are recommendations that non-particulate steroid preparations should be considered as first-line agents when performing ESI [86, 87]. However, further studies are necessary to compare corticosteroid preparations.

Unfortunately, there is no definitive consensus regarding the optimal interval and dosage of ESI. Also, little information concerning recommendations or practice guidelines is available to date. Significant differences were observed in the selection and dose of steroids as well as in the ESI interval. It is mostly attributed to physician preference, who should be aware of the possibility of repeated ESI [88]. We should bear in mind that repeated ESIs within 3 months provide cumulative effects [89]. An appropriate interval between ESIs should be decided based on the average duration of HPA axis suppression after ESI without affecting the physiological restoration. Multiple ESIs using particulate steroids require a sufficient interval of about 3–4 weeks due to a long-lasting HPA axis suppression, while non-particulate steroids require shorter periods. The World Institute of Pain (WIP) Benelux working group recommended that the number of ESIs should be adjusted according to the clinical response, suggesting that a 2-week interval for additional ESI may be appropriate for proper evaluation and minimization of endocrine side effects, and the lowest effective dose should be used for ESI (40 mg for methylprednisolone, 10 to 20 mg for triamcinolone, and 10 mg for dexamethasone) [90].

In the future, determining the optimal steroid dose, duration, and interval for ESIs is essential to develop a treatment protocol with minimal complications without compromising the treatment's effectiveness.

## 6. Adjuvants for epidural administration

In the last few decades, several non-anesthetic applications for epidural procedures have emerged. Epidural catheter infusion techniques of analgesics are being used increasingly for pain control at the end of life in both children and adults, including those with cancer-related pain [91]. In addition to opioids, which are commonly added to epidurally administered local anesthetics, a large number of other pharmacologic agents have been used. Most of these are administered as adjuvants, such as clonidine and dexmedetomidine, while ketamine and neostigmine are still under investigation and are not part of routine clinical practice. Others can be administered as the sole drug, such as antineoplastic drugs (i.e., methotrexate for primary CNS lymphoma) or antibiotics (for ventriculitis or post-neurosurgical infections) [92].

A broad understanding of the pharmacology of those agents is essential for the clinician to utilize them safely and efficiently. Furthermore, it is important to realize that many of those drugs have not been approved for epidural use and are hence used off-label, even when clinically established [93]. **Table 2** reveals the list of Food and Drug Administration (FDA)-approved neuraxial drugs.

### 6.1 Alpha-adrenergic receptor agonists

Alpha-adrenergic receptor agonists are added to neuraxial drugs for several reasons: reducing local anesthetic clearance and distribution from the epidural and spinal space, an intrinsic analgesic effect, and a local anesthetic-sparing property [94]. In this way, complications and side effects associated with the use of epidural local anesthetics and/or opioids can potentially be reduced. Clonidine and dexmedetomidine are the two most important representatives that can cause dose-dependent side effects (sedation, hypotension, and bradycardia) [95]. Therefore, it is important to make a clear risk-benefit assessment before administering any of these drugs neuraxially.

#### *6.1.1 Clonidine*

Clonidine exerts a direct analgesic effect by binding to α2-adrenoceptors in the spinal cord, leading to presynaptic inhibition of Aδ and C-fiber transmitter release. Neuraxial administration of clonidine has a dose-sparing effect on local anesthetics and local anesthetics combined with an opioid, which could reduce the incidence of adverse events [96]. It can produce local vasoconstriction, decreasing the vascular clearance of the local anesthetic around neural structures. It is also a highly lipophilic substance and therefore exerts systemic absorption, with redistribution to more peripheral sites of action [97]. Therefore, adequate hemodynamic monitoring is necessary when administering clonidine to patients.

#### *6.1.2 Dexmedetomidine*

Dexmedetomidine is a selective central α2-adrenergic agonist with sedative properties and works similar to clonidine. When administered as a neuraxial adjuvant, it reduces the required local anesthetic dose and prolongs and potentiates postoperative analgesia [98]. Although the FDA has not approved dexmedetomidine as an adjuvant in neuraxial blocks, it is widely used and is still in use in anesthesia practice as an adjuvant in regional anesthesia for both epidural and intrathecal modalities. In several studies, 1–2 μg/kg of dexmedetomidine along with bupivacaine for caudal epidural block led to prolonged analgesia without significant side effects [99, 100]. Also, dexmedetomidine during labor epidural analgesia demonstrated good maternal satisfaction without deleterious effects on uteroplacental circulation and newborns' outcomes [101]. Nevertheless, there is still insufficient safety data to support the use of neuraxial dexmedetomidine in the clinical setting.

#### *6.1.3 Adrenaline (epinephrine)*

Adrenaline (epinephrine) is used both epidurally and intrathecally to enhance the duration and intensity of neuraxial drugs. It causes vasoconstriction of blood vessels, which reduces neuraxial clearance [94]. Low intrathecal doses (less than 100 μg) led to prolonged sensory and motor block duration but were associated with a greater incidence of hypotension or PONV [102]. Also, neuraxial adrenaline can potentially exacerbate local anesthetic-induced neurotoxic damage in patients whose spinal cord circulation is compromised (such as can occur with diabetes mellitus or arteriosclerosis) [103]. Based on a systematic review, the beneficial effects of adding epidural epinephrine to a local anesthetic remain uncertain [104].

## 6.2 Miscellaneous adjuvants commonly used via epidural route

### *6.2.1 Ketamine*

Ketamine is a selective, non-competitive *N*-methyl-D-aspartate (NMDA) receptor antagonist, with analgesic and anti-hyperalgesic effects. The side effects of ketamine include psychological and mild sympathomimetic effects. There is still no conclusive evidence that epidural ketamine is superior to intravenous administration [105, 106]. Although a systematic review showed a statistically significant, but probably clinically irrelevant, minimal reduction in pain scores when epidural ketamine was used in conjunction with opioids [107].

### *6.2.2 Magnesium*

Magnesium is an NMDA receptor antagonist and regulates the influx of calcium into cells, both resulting in an analgesic effect. Due to the fact that magnesium does not cross the blood-brain barrier easily, it is also used neuraxially [108]. Systematic reviews have shown that epidural administration of magnesium prolongs the time to the first analgesic rescue medication, provides a minimal difference in early pain scores at rest after intrathecal use, and provides a 30% reduction in cumulative morphine use in the first 24 h after surgery [108, 109]. In animal studies, neuraxial magnesium has a neurotoxic potential [110], but to date, no optimal epidural magnesium doses in humans have been established. This should raise caution when one is considering administrating magnesium neuraxial.

### *6.2.3 Midazolam*

Midazolam is a benzodiazepine and is an indirect agonist of gamma-aminobutyric acid (GABA) receptors in the spinal cord. It causes neural inhibition by facilitating the influx of chloride into cells. Epidural administration of midazolam as an adjuvant to local anesthetic in a postoperative continuous infusion increases analgesic and sedative effects and also reduces nausea and vomiting [111, 112]. However, midazolam appears to exacerbate the neurotoxic properties of local anesthetics [113], and therefore, it is questionable if midazolam is appropriate and safe for administration *via* the neuraxial route.

### *6.2.4 Neostigmine*

Neostigmine, a quaternary ammonium salt, is an indirectly acting parasympathomimetic. Inhibition of cholinesterase prolongs and enhances the effect of acetylcholine on muscarinic and nicotinic receptors. Adding neostigmine to epidural morphine increases the time for administration of the first analgesic rescue medication, but total opioid consumption does not change [114, 115]. Neuraxial neostigmine has multiple side effects, including hypotension, sedation, and especially nausea and vomiting, but it does not appear to cause neurotoxicity [115].

| | FDA approval | Epidural | Intrathecal |
|---|---|---|---|
| Local anesthetics | Lidocaine | Yes | Yes |
| | Bupivacaine | Yes | Yes |
| | Levobupivacaine | Yes | No |
| | Ropivacaine | Yes | No |
| | Mepivacaine | Yes | No |
| | Chloroprocaine | Yes | Yes |
| | Tetracaine | No | No |
| Opioids | Morphine | Yes | Yes |
| | Sufentanil | Yes | Yes |
| | Fentanyl | No | Yes |
| | Hydromorphone | No | No |
| | Buprenorphine | No | No |
| | Diamorphine | No | No |
| | Tramadol | No | No |
| | Methadone | No | No |
| | Meperidine | No | No |
| | Levorphanol | No | No |
| | Butorphanol | No | No |
| | Oxymorphone | No | No |
| | Pentazocine | No | No |
| Calcium channel antagonists | Ziconotide | No | Yes |
| | Gabapentin | No | No |
| | Verapamil | No | No |
| GABA agonists | Baclofen | No | Yes |
| | Muscimol | No | No |
| | Midazolam | No | No |
| Cyclooxygenase inhibitors | Ketorolac | No | No |
| | Aspirin | No | No |
| | Perecoxib | No | No |
| | Lornoxicam | No | No |
| Cholinergic agonists | Neostigmine | No | No |
| Adenosine agonists | Adenosine | No | No |
| Dopamine antagonists | Droperidol | No | No |
| Corticosteroids | Methylprednisolone | No | No |
| | Hydrocortisone | No | No |
| | Triamcinolone | No | No |
| | Betamethasone | No | No |
| | Dexamethasone | No | No |

| | FDA approval | Epidural | Intrathecal |
|---|---|---|---|
| NMDA receptor antagonists | Ketamine | No | No |
| | Esketamine | No | No |
| Somatostatin agonists | Octreotide | No | No |
| Adrenergic agonists | Clonidine | Yes | No |
| | Dexmedetomidine | No | No |
| | Adrenaline (epinephrine) | No | No |
| | Epinephrine co-administered with bupivacaine | Yes | No |
| | Epinephrine co-administered with lidocaine | Yes | No |
| | Phenylephrine | No | No |
| Adjuvants | Magnesium sulfate | No | No |
| | Sodium bicarbonate | No | No |
| | Dextran | No | No |

**Table 6.**
*FDA US Food and Drug Administration, GABA gamma-aminobutyric acid, NMDA N-methyl-D-aspartate [91].*

The use of adjuvants with LAs has been practiced for many years and remains the subject of much interest. Many anesthesiologists advocate their use since their nomination with LAs allows the reduction in doses of both classes of drugs, thus lessening the likelihood of side effects attributed to each. Although the evidence for significant benefit is limited (i.e., clonidine or adrenaline), other adjuvants have been found to be effective but at the expense of frequent side effects (i.e., neostigmine). At this point, only the role of NMDA receptor antagonists seems favorable, and further studies are awaited. Furthermore, many of those drugs have not been approved for neuraxial use and are hence used off-label, partially due to the lack of large clinical trials. Therefore, it is important to make a clear risk-benefit assessment before epidural administration of any of these drugs (**Table 6**).

## 7. Future perspectives

In addition to the currently approved drugs for neuraxial administration, a whole range of new drugs has been approved for other indications or routes of administration, but are still used off-label for spinal or epidural injections.

As for local anesthetics are concerned, some of the old agents have been reinforced, such as **2-chloroprocaine** [116] and **prilocaine** [117]. Both of them are used for short-duration spinal anesthesia and have a promising place in day-case surgery. However, both of them are still not approved for epidural administration (**Table 1**). Also, novel long-lasting LAs have been developed. **Tonicaine (n-β-phenylethyl lidocaine)** [118] and **n-butyl-tetracaine** [119], derivatives of lidocaine and tetracaine, produce prolonged sensory blockade, which lasts longer than motor blockade, and the onset of action is significantly slower than with the original agent. Another LA that has shown promise as a long-acting agent is **n-butyl amino-benzoate** (BAB) [120, 121]. A single epidural or peripheral nerve block using BAB has provided pain relief for up to 14 weeks, and it has been used successfully in the management of excruciating pain associated with advanced malignancy. It provides good and long-lasting analgesia combined with a low incidence of motor blockade. Future studies are required to establish the safety of these LAs.

A variety of **animal toxins** such as tetrodotoxin (a naturally occurring toxin of the puffer fish fugu), ProTx-II peptide (from the venom of the tarantula), or omega-conotoxin (from the venom of piscivorous marine snails) specifically block voltage-sensitive calcium channels in a way similar to LAs [122, 123], but their clinical use is still limited due to considerable systemic toxicity.

Some previously established drugs have been found to have LAs effects: **Sameridine** and **pethidine** are compounds with LA and opioid actions, which have been used successfully as intrathecal agents in human studies. The duration of a sensory blockade is similar to that of lidocaine, but analgesia is more prolonged and without side effects such as respiratory depression [124, 125]. **Tricyclic antidepressants** (such as amitriptyline) share several properties, both physical and pharmacological, with LAs. They share a common mechanism of action with both blocking neuronal sodium channels in a use-dependent manner, although tricyclic antidepressants also affect numerous other neurotransmitters including serotonin, glutamate, adenosine, and acetylcholine [126].

Additionally, **advances in delivery systems** have been made. The liposomal delivery system has been developed in an attempt to prolong the duration of action of administered LAs without the need for adjuvant drugs, nerve sheath catheters or pumps. Liposomes are microscopic lipid vesicles (0.02–40 μm) that act as a reservoir of drugs. They prevent redistribution from the site of injection to other tissues, due to the fact that a very small fraction of the drug is bioavailable and therefore, decreases the risk of systemic toxicity. Work in animal models and in humans has shown that the release of liposomal-encapsulated LAs and morphine occurs more slowly than with standard preparations of either drug, resulting in a prolonged analgesic effect without an increase in the time to onset of analgesia [127, 128]. Improved pain scores and decreased opioid consumption have been demonstrated for up to 48 h after lower abdominal surgery, hip arthroplasty, and Cesarean section [129–131]. The safety of liposomal preparations is yet to be fully established. There are concerns regarding the potential neurotoxicity of the liposomes and a risk for liposomal breakdown, resulting in the rapid release of large amounts of free drugs [132]. Hopefully, in the future, these delivery systems should provide the clinician with both an extended range and a choice in the degree of prolongation of the action of each agent.

## 8. Conclusion

Epidural anesthesia and analgesia often present as a supplement to general anesthesia for surgical procedures in pediatric and adult patients. Medications administrated in epidural space provide analgesia in intraoperative, postoperative, peripartum, and end-of-life settings with a special benefit in a group of elderly patients and those with different comorbidities. Special caution is required during the procedure since the epidural space is “virtual” with anatomical relationships and possible spine pathology that makes the epidural space irregular and segmental, and can affect the spread of the medications and their final drug efficacy. The main goal of the epidural blockade is to produce a quality sensory block with the lack of motor block. However, autonomic fibers are more susceptible to blockade and reach 2–6 dermatomal levels higher than the sensory block, resulting in cardiovascular and hemodynamic changes that affect almost all organ systems, respectively.

Drugs administrated in the epidural space pass their way to the site of action by diffusion into the CSF through the spinal meninges and are influenced by dose, volume, and concentration of the drug, surface area, protein binding, and lipid solubility, respectively. LAs in a combination with opioids are the most common epidural administrated drugs. LAs inhibit action potential in nociceptive fibers and block the transmission of pain impulses by blocking VGSC. By duration of action, they are classified into the short-, intermediate-, and long-acting groups. On the other hand, opioids are lipid-soluble weak bases that are highly bound to the proteins and are ionized at physiologic pH. They bind to four main types of opioid receptors mainly located in the dorsal horn of the spinal cord, each having their prototype agonist producing the clinical effect. Special caution must be set on their adverse effects with an emphasis on the life-threatening event called local anesthetic systemic toxicity (LAST) and opioid-related depression of the ventilation, that must be treated timely.

New treatment techniques for patients suffering from back pain syndrome include epidural steroid injection (ESI) with corticosteroid administration into the epidural space having an anti-inflammatory effect. Corticosteroids can have a severity of complications. Therefore, a 2-week interval for additional ESI is suggested. Dexamethasone is considered generally safer than methylprednisolone, but further studies are necessary. In addition to the mentioned drugs, many other drugs can help in achieving a successful epidural block, such as adjuvants. However, many of them have not been approved for epidural use and hence are used off-label, even when clinically established. Additionally, new LAs, animal toxins, and liposomal delivery systems have been developed in an attempt to provide clinically effective epidural block.

Since epidural blockade is a complex process, which takes place at many different sites, further investigations are required to fill the gaps in our knowledge of the fundamental process of epidural action. The majority of variables involved in epidural drug efficacy are not susceptible to direct measurement. Therefore, careful experimental design and examination of direct and indirect evidence from clinical and laboratory sources are needed for better clarification.

## Conflict of interest

The authors declare no conflict of interest.

## Author details

Katarina Tomulić Brusich[1*], Lara Valenčić[1,2] and Željka Polonijo[1]

1 Department of Anesthesiology, Intensive Medicine and Pain Treatment, Clinical Hospital Centre Rijeka, Rijeka, Croatia

2 Faculty of Medicine, University of Rijeka, Rijeka, Croatia

*Address all correspondence to: ktomulic@gmail.com

## References

[1] Bauer M, George JE 3rd, Seif J. Recent advances in epidural analgesia. Anesthesiology and Research Practice. 2012;**2012**:309219. DOI: 10.1155/2012/309219

[2] Schnabel A, Thyssen NM, Goeters C. Age- and procedure-specific differences of epidural analgesia in children--a database analysis. Pain Medicine. 2015;**16**(3):544-553. DOI: 10.1111/pme.12633

[3] Licker M, Schweizer A, Ellenberger C. Perioperative medical management of patients with COPD. International Journal of Chronic Obstructive Pulmonary Disease. 2007;**2**(4):493-515

[4] Eyelade O, Sanusi A, Adigun T. Outcome of anesthesia in elective surgical patients with comorbidities. Annals of African Medicine. 2016;**15**(2):78-82. DOI: 10.4103/1596-3519.176204

[5] Kojima Y, Narita M. Postoperative outcome among elderly patients after general anesthesia. Acta Anaesthesiologica Scandinavica. 2006;**50**(1):19-25. DOI: 10.1111/j.1399-6576.2005.00882.x

[6] Manion SC, Brennan TJ, Riou B. Thoracic epidural analgesia and acute pain management. Anesthesiology. 2011;**115**(1):181-188. DOI: 10.1097/ALN.0b013e318220847c

[7] Wuethrich PY, Hsu Schmitz SF, Kessler TM. Potential influence of the anesthetic technique used during open radical prostatectomy on prostate cancer-related outcome: A retrospective study. Anesthesiology. 2010;**113**(3):570-576. DOI: 10.1097/ALN.0b013e3181e4f6ec

[8] Liu D, Sun C, Zhang X. Influence of epidural anesthesia and general anesthesia on thromboembolism in patients undergoing total knee arthroplasty. American Journal of Translational Research. 2021;**13**(9):10933-10941 eCollection 2021

[9] Park WY, Thompson JS, Lee KK. Effect of epidural anesthesia and analgesia on perioperative outcome: A randomized, controlled veterans affairs cooperative study. Annals of Surgery. 2001;**234**(4):560-569; discussion 569-571. DOI: 10.1097/00000658-200110000-00015

[10] Bromage PR. The physiology and pharmacology of epidural blockade. Clinical Anesthesia. 1969;**2**:45-61

[11] Savolaine ER, Pandya JB, Greenblatt SH. Anatomy of the human lumbar epidural space: New insights using CT- epidurography. Anesthesiology. 1988;**68**(2):217-220. DOI: 10.1097/00000542-198802000-00007

[12] Macpherson D, Quondamatteo F, Broom M. Update on applied epidural anatomy. BJA Education. 2022;**22**(5):182-189. DOI: 10.1016/j.bjae.2021.12.006

[13] Hogan QH. Lumbar epidural anatomy. A new look by cryomicrotome section. Anesthesiology. 1991;**75**(5):767-775. DOI: 10.1097/00000542-199111000-00007

[14] Igarashi T, Hirabayashi Y, Shimizu R. The lumbar extradural structure changes with increasing age. British Journal of Anaesthesia. 1997;**78**(2):149-152. DOI: 10.1093/bja/78.2.149

[15] Arendt K, Segal S. Why epidurals do not always work. Reviews in Obstetrics and Gynecology. 2008;**1**(2):49-55

[16] Maddali P, Moisi M, Page J. Anatomical complications of epidural anesthesia: A comprehensive review. Clinical Anatomy. 2017;**30**(3):342-346. DOI: 10.1002/ca.22831

[17] White JL, Stevens RA, Kao TC. Differential sensory block: Spinal vs epidural with lidocaine. Canadian Journal of Anaesthesia. 1998;**45**(11):1049-1053. DOI: 10.1007/BF03012390

[18] Taylor A, McLeod G. Basic pharmacology of local anesthetics. BJA Education. 2020;**20**(2):34-41. DOI: 10.1016/j.bjae.2019.10.002

[19] Rizk MK, Tolba R, Kapural L. Differential epidural block predicts the success of visceral block in patients with chronic visceral abdominal pain. Pain Practice. 2012;**12**(8):595-601. DOI: 10.1111/J.1533-2500.2012.00548.x

[20] Colvin LA. Physiology and pharmacology of pain. In: Thompson JP, Wiles MD, Moppett IG, editors. Smith and Aitkenhead's Textbook of Anesthesia. 7th ed. St Louis: Elsevier; 2019. pp. 100-121

[21] Hodgson PS, Liu SS. Epidural lidocaine decreases sevoflurane requirement for adequate depth of anesthesia as measured by the Bispectral index monitor. Anesthesiology. 2001;**94**(5):799-803. DOI: 10.1097/00000542-200105000-00018

[22] Clemente A, Carli F. The physiological effects of thoracic epidural anesthesia and analgesia on the cardiovascular, respiratory and gastrointestinal systems. Minerva Anestesiologica. 2008;**74**(10):549-563

[23] Groeben H. Epidural anesthesia and pulmonary function. Journal of Anesthesia. 2006;**20**(4):290-299. DOI: 10.1007/s00540-006-0425-6

[24] van Lier F, van der Geest PJ, Hoeks SE. Epidural analgesia is associated with improved health outcomes of surgical patients with chronic obstructive pulmonary disease. Anesthesiology. 2011;**115**(2):315-321. DOI: 10.1097/ALN.0b013e318224cc5c

[25] Moraca RJ, Sheldon DG, Thirlby RC. The role of epidural anesthesia and analgesia in surgical practice. Annals of Surgery. 2003;**238**(5):663-673. DOI: 10.1097/01.sla.0000094300.36689.ad

[26] Suleiman MY, Passannante AN, Onder RL. Alteration of renal blood flow during epidural anesthesia in normal subjects. Anesthesia and Analgesia. 1997;**84**(5):1076-1080. DOI: 10.1097/00000539-199705000-00022

[27] Wu Z, Zhu Y. Comparison of the effects of epidural anesthesia and general anesthesia on perioperative cognitive function and deep vein thrombosis in patients undergoing Total knee arthroplasty. Evidence-based Complementary and Alternative Medicine. 2021;**2021**:1565067. DOI: 10.1155/2021/1565067

[28] Yaksh TL, Fisher CJ, Hockman TM. Current and future issues in the development of spinal agents for the management of pain. Current Neuropharmacology. 2017;**15**(2):232-259. DOI: 10.2174/1570159x14666160307145542

[29] Bromage PR, Burfoot MF. Quality of epidural blockade. II. Influence of physico-chemical factors; hyaluronidase and potassium. British Journal of Anaesthesia. 1966;**38**(11):857-865. DOI: 10.1093/bja/38.11.857

[30] Visser WA, Lee RA, Gielen MJM. Factors affecting the distribution of a neural blockade by local anesthetics in epidural anesthesia and a comparison of lumbar versus thoracic epidural anesthesia. Anesthesia and Analgesia. 2008;**107**(2):708-721. DOI: 10.1213/ane.0b013e31817e7065

[31] NYSORA. The New York School of Regional Anesthesia. Epidural Anesthesia and Analgesia [Internet]. 2022. Available from: https://www.nysora.com/topics/regional-anesthesia-for-specific-surgical-procedures/abdomen/epidural-anesthesia-analgesia/#toc_PHARMACOLOGY-OF-EPIDURAL-block. [Accessed: September 30, 2022]

[32] Stoelting RK, Hillier SC. Local anesthetics. In: Stoelting RK, Hillier SC, editors. Handbook of Pharmacology & Physiology in Anesthetic Practice. 2nd ed. Philadelphia: Lippincott Williams & Wilkins; 2006. pp. 179-188

[33] Becker DE, Reed KL. Essentials of local anesthetic pharmacology. Anesthesia Prof. 2006;**53**(3):98-109. DOI: 10.2344/0003-3006(2006)53[98,EOLAP]2.0.CO;2

[34] Lirk P, Picardi S, Hollmann MW. Local anaesthetics: 10 essentials. European Journal of Anaesthesiology. 2014;**31**(11):575-585. DOI: 10.1097/EJA.0000000000000137

[35] Lirk P, Hollmann MW, Strichartz G. The science of local anesthesia: Basic research, clinical application, and future directions. Anesthesia and Analgesia. 2018;**126**(4):1381-1392. DOI: 10.1213/ANE.0000000000002665

[36] Ogura T, Egan TD. Opioid agonists and antagonists. In: Hemmings H, Talmage E, editors. Pharmacology and Physiology for Anesthesia: Foundations and Clinical Application. 1st ed. Philadelphia: Elsevier Saunders; 2013. pp. 253-271

[37] Corder G, Castro D, Bruchas M. Endogenous and exogenous opioids in pain. Annual Review of Neuroscience. 2018;**41**(1):453-473. DOI: 10.1146/annurev-neuro-080317-061522

[38] Bernards C, Shen D, Sterling E. Epidural, cerebrospinal fluid, and plasma pharmacokinetics of epidural opioids (part 1). Anesthesiology. 2003;**99**(2):455-465. DOI: 10.1097/00000542-200308000-00029

[39] Bernards C, Shen D, Sterling E. Epidural, cerebrospinal fluid, and plasma pharmacokinetics of epidural opioids (part 2). Anesthesiology. 2003;**99**(2):466-475. DOI: 10.1097/00000542-200308000-00030

[40] Coda B, Brown M, Schaffer R. Pharmacology of epidural fentanyl, alfentanil, and sufentanil in volunteers. Anesthesiology. 1994;**81**(5):1149-1161. DOI: 10.1097/00000542-199411000-00008

[41] Ummenhofer WC, Arends RH, Shen DD. Comparative spinal distribution and clearance kinetics of intrathecally administered morphine, fentanyl, alfentanil, and sufentanil. Anesthesiology. 2000;**92**(3):739-753. DOI: 10.1097/00000542-200003000-00018

[42] Congedo E, Sgreccia M, De Cosmo G. New drugs for epidural analgesia. Current Drug Targets. 2009;**10**(8):696-706. DOI: 10.2174/138945009788982441

[43] Bujedo BM, Santos SG, Azpiazu AU. A review of epidural and intrathecal opioids used in the management of postoperative pain. Journal of Opioid

Management. 2012;**8**(3):177-192. DOI: 10.5055/jom.2012.0114

[44] Jiang X, Wen X, Gao B. The plasma concentrations of lidocaine after slow versus rapid administration of an initial dose of epidural anesthesia. Anesthesia and Analgesia. 1997;**84**(3):570-573

[45] Rose FX, Estebe JP, Ratajczak M. Epidural, intrathecal pharmacokinetics, and intrathecal bioavailability of ropivacaine. Anesthesia and Analgesia. 2007;**105**(3):859-867. DOI: 10.1213/01.ane.0000278129.37099.fa

[46] Bromage PR. Spread of analgesic solutions in the epidural space and their site of action: A statistical study. British Journal of Anaesthesia. 1962;**34**:161-178. DOI: 10.1093/bja/34.3.161

[47] Veering BT, Burm AG, Vletter AA. The effect of age on the systemic absorption, disposition and pharmacodynamics of bupivacaine after epidural administration. Clinical Pharmacokinetics. 1992;**22**(1):75-84. DOI: 10.2165/00003088-199222010-00007

[48] Berde CB, Koka A, Drasner K. Local anesthetics. In: Pardo MC Jr, Miller RD, editors. Basics of Anesthesia. 7th ed. Elsevier; 2018. pp. 150-151

[49] Panni MK, Columb MO. Obese parturients have lower epidural local anaesthetic requirements for analgesia in labour. British Journal of Anaesthesia. 2006;**96**(1):106-110. DOI: 10.1093/bja/aei284

[50] Moller RA, Covino BG. Effect of progesterone on the cardiac electrophysiologic alterations produced by ropivacaine and bupivacaine. Anesthesiology. 1992;**77**(4):735-741. DOI: 10.1097/00000542-199210000-00018

[51] Bromage PR, Joyal AC, Binney JC. Local anesthetic drugs: Penetration from the spinal extradural space into the neuraxis. Science. 1963;**140**(3565):392-394. DOI: 10.1126/science.140.3565.392

[52] Li Y, Cong H, Fan Y. Epidural analgesia with amide local anesthetics, bupivacaine, and ropivacaine in combination with fentanyl for labor pain relief: A meta-analysis. Medical Science Monitor. 2015;**21**:921-928. DOI: 10.12659/MSM.892276

[53] Becker DE, Reed KL. Local anesthetics: Review of pharmacological considerations. Anesthesia Progress. 2012;**59**(2):90-102. DOI: 10.2344/0003-3006-59.2.90

[54] Tonder S, Togioka BM, Maani CV. Chloroprocaine. StatPearls Publishing; 2022

[55] Beecham GB, Nessel TA, Goyal A. Lidocaine. StatPearls Publishing; 2021

[56] Beilin Y, Halpern S. Focused review: Ropivacaine versus bupivacaine for epidural labor analgesia. Anesthesia and Analgesia. 2010;**111**(2):482-487. DOI: 10.1213/ANE.0b013e3181e3a08e

[57] Bajwa SJS, Kaur J. Clinical profile of levobupivacaine in regional anesthesia: A systematic review. Journal of Anaesthesiology Clinical Pharmacology. 2013;**29**(4):530-539. DOI: 10.4103/0970-9185.119172

[58] Shipton EA. New formulations of local anaesthetics – Part I. Anesthesiology and Research Practice. 2012;**2012**:546409. DOI: 10.1155/2012/546409

[59] Kuthiala G, Chaudhary G. Ropivacaine: A review of its pharmacology and clinical use. Indian Journal of Anaesthesia.

2011;**55**(2):104-110. DOI: 10.4103/0019-5049.79875

[60] El-Boghdadly K, Pawa A, Chin KJ. Local anesthetic systemic toxicity:Current perspectives. Local and Regional Anesthesia. 2018;**11**:35-44. DOI: 10.2147/LRA.S154512

[61] Sepulveda EA, Pak A. Lipid Emulsion Therapy. StatPearls Publishing; 2022

[62] American Society of Regional Anesthesia and Pain Medicine. Checklist for treatment of local anesthetic toxicity. Available from: https://www.asra.com/docs/default-source/guidelines-articles/local-anesthetic-systemic-toxicity-rgb.pdf?sfvrsn=33b348e_2. [Accessed: September 30, 2022]

[63] Trescot A, Datta S, Lee M. Opioid pharmacology. Pain Physician. 2008;**11**(2Suppl):S133-S153

[64] Dhaliwal A, Gupta M. Physiology, Opioid Receptor. StatPearls Publishing; 2022

[65] McDonald J, Lambert D. Opioid receptors. BJA Education. 2015;**15**(5):219-224. DOI: 10.1093/bjaceaccp/mku041

[66] Chaney M. Side effects of intrathecal and epidural opioids. Canadian Journal of Anaesthesia. 1995;**42**(10):891-903. DOI: 10.1007/BF03011037

[67] Aldrete J. Reduction of nausea and vomiting from epidural opioids by adding droperidol to the infusate in home-bound patients. Journal of Pain and Symptom Management. 1995;**10**(7):544-547. DOI: 10.1016/0885-3924(95)00104-7

[68] Beeby D, MacIntosh KC, Bailey M. Postoperative analgesia for caesarean section using epidural methadone. Anaesthesia. 1984;**39**(1):61-63. DOI: 10.1111/j.1365-2044.1984.tb09459.x

[69] Welch DB, Hrynaszkiewicz A. Postoperative analgesia using epidural methadone. Administration by the lumbar route for thoracic pain relief. Anaesthesia. 1981;**36**(11):1051-1054. DOI: 10.1111/j.1365-2044.1981.tb08681.x

[70] Elbaridi N, Kaye AD, Choi S. Current concepts of Phenylpiperidine derivatives use in the treatment of acute and chronic pain. Pain Physician. 2017;**20**(2):SE23-SE31

[71] Grass JA. Sufentanil: Clinical use as postoperative analgesic—Epidural/intrathecal route. Journal of Pain and Symptom Management. 1992;**7**(5):271-286. DOI: 10.1016/0885-3924(92)90061-l

[72] Stanislaus MA, Reno JL, Small RH. Continuous epidural hydromorphone infusion for post-cesarean delivery analgesia in a patient on methadone maintenance therapy: A case report. Journal of Pain Research. 2020;**13**:837-842. DOI: 10.2147/JPR.S242271

[73] Piirainen P, Kokki H, Kokki M. Epidural oxycodone for acute pain. Pharmaceuticals (Basel). 2022;**15**(5):643. DOI: 10.3390/ph15050643

[74] Piirainen P, Kokki H, Anderson B. Analgesic efficacy and pharmacokinetics of epidural oxycodone in pain management after gynaecological laparoscopy—A randomised, double blind, active control, double-dummy clinical comparison with intravenous administration. British Journal of Clinical Pharmacology. 2019;**85**(8):1798-1807. DOI: 10.1111/bcp.13971

[75] Bicket MC, Horowitz JM, Benzon HT. Epidural injections in prevention of surgery for spinal pain: Systematic review and meta-analysis of randomized

controlled trials. The Spine Journal. 2015;**15**(2):348-362. DOI: 10.1016/j.spinee.2014.10.011

[76] Collighan N, Gupta S. Epidural steroids. Continuing Education in Anaesthesia Critical Care & Pain. 2010;**10**(1):1-5. DOI: 10.1093/bjaceaccp/mkp043

[77] Boden SD, Davis DO, Dina TS. Abnormal magnetic-resonance scans of the lumbar spine in asymp- tomatic subjects. A prospective investigation. The Journal of Bone and Joint Surgery. American Volume. 1990;**72**:403-408

[78] McLain RF, Kapural L, Mekhail NA. Epidural steroid therapy for back and leg pain: Mechanisms of action and efficacy. The Spine Journal. 2005;**5**:191-201. DOI: 10.1016/j.spinee.2004.10.046

[79] Friedly JL, Comstock BA, Heagerty PJ. Systemic effects of epidural steroid injections for spinal stenosis. Pain. 2018;**159**:876-883

[80] Guyatt G, Gutterman D, Baumann MH. Grading strength of recommendations and quality of evidence in clinical guidelines: Report from an American College of Chest Physician task force. Chest. 2006;**129**(1):174-181. DOI: 10.1378/chest.129.1.174

[81] Nelson DA, Landau WM. Intraspinal steroids: History, efficacy, accidentality, and controversy with review of United States Food and Drug Administration reports. Journal of Neurology, Neurosurgery, and Psychiatry. 2001;**70**(4):433-443. DOI: 10.1136/jnnp.70.4.433

[82] Manchikanti L, Rajgopal RP, Pampati V. Comparison of three routes of epidural steroid injections in low back pain. Pain Digest. 1999;**9**:277-285

[83] Sim SE, Hong HJ, Roh K. Relationship between epidural steroid dose and suppression of hypothalamus-pituitary-adrenal axis. Pain Physician. 2020;**23**(4S):S283-S294

[84] Houten JK, Errico TJ. Paraplegia after lumbosacral nerve root block: Report of three cases. The Spine Journal. 2002;**2**:70-75. DOI: 10.1016/s1529-9430(01)00159-0

[85] Derby R, Lee S-H, Date ES. Size and aggregation of corticosteroids used for epidural injections. Pain Medicine. 2008;**9**(2):227-234. DOI: 10.1111/j.1526-4637.2007.00341.x

[86] Donohue NK, Tarima SS, Durand MJ. Comparing pain relief and functional improvement between methylpredniso-lone and dexamethasone lumbosacral transforaminal epidural steroid injections: A self-controlled study. Korean J Pain. 2020;**33**:192-198. DOI: 10.3344/kjp.2020.33.2.192

[87] Vydra D, McCormick Z, Clements N. Current trends in steroid dose choice and frequency of Administration of Epidural Steroid Injections: A survey study. PM & R : The Journal of Injury, Function, and Rehabilitation. 2020;**12**(1):49-54. DOI: 10.1002/pmrj.12192

[88] Kim EJ, Moon JY, Park KS. Epidural steroid injection in Korean pain physicians: A national survey. Korean J Pain. 2014;**27**(1):35-42. DOI: 10.3344/kjp.2014.27.1.35

[89] Murthy NS, Geske JR, Shelerud RA. The effectiveness of repeat lumbar transforaminal epidural steroid injections. Pain Medicine. 2014;**15**(10):1686-1694. DOI: 10.1111/pme.12497

[90] Van Boxem K, Rijsdijk M, Hans G. Safe use of epidural corticosteroid

injections: Recommendations of the WIP Benelux work group. Pain Practice. 2019;**19**:61-92. DOI: 10.1111/papr.12709

[91] Hermanns H, Bos EME, van Zuylen ML. The options for Neuraxial drug administration. CNS Drugs. 2022;**36**(8):877-896. DOI: 10.1007/s40263-022-00936-y

[92] Prabhakar A, Lambert T, Kaye RJ. Adjuvants in clinical regional anesthesia practice: A comprehensive review. Best Practice & Research. Clinical Anaesthesiology. 2019;**33**(4):415-423. DOI: 10.1016/j.bpa.2019.06.001

[93] van Zuylen ML, Hoope WT, Bos E. Safety of epidural drugs: A narrative review. Expert Opinion on Drug Safety. 2019;**18**(7):591-601. DOI: 10.1080/14740338.2019.1617271

[94] Niemi G, Breivik H. Epinephrine markedly improves thoracic epidural analgesia produced by a small-dose infusion of ropivacaine, fentanyl, and epinephrine after major surgery: A randomized, double-blinded crossover study with and without epinephrine. Anesthesia and Analgesia. 2002;**94**(6):1598-1605. DOI: 10.1213/00000539-200206000-00044

[95] De Kock M, Wiederkher P, Laghmiche A. Epidural clonidine used as the sole analgesic agent during and after abdominal surgery: A dose-response study. Anesthesiology. 1997;**86**(2):285-292. DOI: 10.1097/00000542-199702000-00003

[96] Rhee K, Kang K, Kim J. Intravenous clonidine prolongs bupivacaine spinal anesthesia. Acta Anaesthesiologica Scandinavica. 2003;**47**(8):1001-1005. DOI: 10.1034/j.1399-6576.2003.00158.x

[97] Jarrott B, Conway EL, Maccarrone C. Clonidine: Understanding its disposition, sites and mechanism of action. Clinical and Experimental Pharmacology & Physiology. 1987;**14**(5):471-479. DOI: 10.1111/j.1440-1681.1987.tb00999.x

[98] Solanki SL, Goyal VK. Neuraxial dexmedetomidine: Wonder drug or simply harmful. Anesthesia and Pain Medicine. 2015;**5**(2):e22651. DOI: 10.5812/aapm.22651

[99] El-Hennawy AM, Abd-Elwahab AM, Abd-Elmaksoud AM. Addition of clonidine or dexmedetomidine to bupivacaine prolongs caudal analgesia in children. British Journal of Anaesthesia. 2009;**103**(2):268-274. DOI: 10.1093/bja/aep159

[100] Elhakim M, Abdelhamid D, Abdelfattach H. Effect of epidural dexmedetomidine on intraoperative awareness and post-operative pain after one-lung ventilation. Acta Anaesthesiologica Scandinavica. 2010;**54**(6):703-709. DOI: 10.1111/j.1399-6576.2009.02199.x

[101] Selim MF, Elnabtity AM, Hasan AM. Comparative evaluation of epidural bupivacaine - dexmedetomidine and bupivacaine -fentanyl on Doppler velocimetry of uterine and umbilical arteries during labor. J Prenat Med. 2012;**6**(3):47-54

[102] de Oliveira GS, Jr BB, Nader A. Dose-ranging effects of intrathecal epinephrine on anesthesia/analgesia: A meta-analysis and metaregression of randomized controlled trials. Regional Anesthesia and Pain Medicine. 2012;**37**(4):423-432. DOI: 10.1097/AAP.0b013e318251fce1

[103] Neal JM. Effects of epinephrine in local anesthetics on the central and peripheral nervous systems: Neurotoxicity and neural blood flow. Regional Anesthesia and Pain Medicine.

2003;**28**(2):124-134. DOI: 10.1053/rapm.2003.50024

[104] Tschopp C, Tramer MR, Schneider A. Benefit and harm of adding epinephrine to a local anesthetic for neuraxial and locoregional anesthesia: A meta-analysis of randomized controlled trials with trial sequential analyses. Anesthesia and Analgesia. 2018;**127**(1):228-239. DOI: 10.1213/ANE.0000000000003417

[105] Tena B, Gomar C, Rios J. Perioperative epidural or intravenous ketamine does not improve the effectiveness of thoracic epidural analgesia for acute and chronic pain after thoracotomy. The Clinical Journal of Pain. 2014;**30**(6):490-500. DOI: 10.1097/AJP.0000000000000005

[106] Xie H, Wang X, Liu G. Analgesic effects and pharmacokinetics of a low dose of ketamine preoperatively administered epidurally or intravenously. The Clinical Journal of Pain. 2003;**19**(5):317-322. DOI: 10.1097/00002508-200309000-00006

[107] Subramaniam K, Subramaniam B, Steinbrook RA. Ketamine as adjuvant analgesic to opioids: A quantitative and qualitative systematic review. Anesthesia and Analgesia. 2004;**99**(2):482-495. DOI: 10.1213/01.ANE.0000118109.12855.07

[108] Albrecht E, Kirkham KR, Liu SS. The analgesic efficacy and safety of neuraxial magnesium sulphate: A quantitative review. Anaesthesia. 2013;**68**(2):190-202. DOI: 10.1111/j.1365-2044.2012.07337.x

[109] Pascual-Ramírez J, Gil-Trujillo S, Alcantarilla C. Intrathecal magnesium as analgesic adjuvant for spinal anesthesia: A meta-analysis of randomized trials. Minerva Anestesiologica. 2013;**79**(6):667-678

[110] Goodman EJ, Haas AJ, Kantor GS. Inadvertent administration of magnesium sulfate through the epidural catheter: Report and analysis of a drug error. International Journal of Obstetric Anesthesia. 2006;**15**(1):63-67. DOI: 10.1016/j.ijoa.2005.06.009

[111] Nishiyama T, Matsukawa T, Hanaoka K. Continuous epidural administration of midazolam and bupivacaine for postoperative analgesia. Acta Anaesthesiologica Scandinavica. 1999;**43**(5):568-572. DOI: 10.1034/j.1399-6576.1999.430514.x

[112] Nishiyama T, Matsukawa T, Hanaoka K. Effects of adding midazolam on the postoperative epidural analgesia with two different doses of bupivacaine. Journal of Clinical Anesthesia. 2002;**14**(2):92-97. DOI: 10.1016/S0952-8180(01)00347-6

[113] Werdehausen R, Braun S, Hermanns H. The influence of adjuvants used in regional anesthesia on lidocaine-induced neurotoxicity in vitro. Regional Anesthesia and Pain Medicine. 2011;**36**(5):436-443. DOI: 10.1097/AAP.0b013e318226ba62

[114] Lauretti GR. The evolution of spinal/epidural neostigmine in clinical application: Thoughts after two decades. Saudi Journal of Anaesthesia. 2015;**9**(1):71-81. DOI: 10.4103/1658-354X.146319

[115] Omais M, Lauretti GR, Paccola CA. Epidural morphine and neostigmine for postoperative analgesia after orthopedic surgery. Anesthesia and Analgesia. 2002;**95**(6):1698-1701. DOI: 10.1097/00000539-200212000-00042

[116] Casati A, Fanelli G, Danelli G. Spinal anesthesia with lidocaine or preservative-free 2-chlorprocaine for outpatient knee arthroscopy: A prospective, randomized, double-blind comparison. Anesthesia and Analgesia. 2007;**104**(4):959-964. DOI: 10.1213/01.ane.0000258766.73612.d8

[117] Ostgaard G, Hallaraker O, Ulveseth OK. A randomised study of lidocaine and prilocaine for spinal anaesthesia. Acta Anaesthesiologica Scandinavica. 2000;**44**(4):436-440. DOI: 10.1034/j.1399-6576.2000.440413.x

[118] Khan MA, Gerner P, Sudoh Y. Use of a charged lidocaine derivative, tonicaine, for prolonged infiltration anesthesia. Regional Anesthesia and Pain Medicine. 2002;**27**(2):173-179. DOI: 10.1053/rapm.2002.28710

[119] Wang GK, Vladimirov M, Quan C. N-butyl tetracaine as a neurolytic agent for ultralong sciatic nerve block. Anesthesiology. 1996;**85**(6):1386-1394. DOI: 10.1097/00000542-199612000-00020

[120] Shulman M. Treatment of cancer pain with epidural butyl-amino-benzoate suspension. Regional Anesthesia. 1987;**12**:1-4. DOI: 10.1136/rapm-00115550-198712010-00001

[121] Grouls RJ, Meert TF, Korsten HH. Epidural and intrathecal n-butyl-p-aminobenzoate solution in the rat. Comparison with bupivacaine. Anesthesiology. 1997;**86**(1):181-187. DOI: 10.1097/00000542-199701000-00022

[122] Schmalhofer WA, Calhoun J, Burrows R. ProTx-II, a selective inhibitor of NaV1.7 sodium channels, blocks action potential propagation in nociceptors. Molecular Pharmacology. 2008;**74**(5):1476-1484. DOI. 10.1124/mol.108.047670

[123] Bowersox S, Gadbois T, Singh T. Selective N-type neuronal voltage-sensitive calcium channel blocker, SNX-111, produces spinal antinociception in rat models of acute, persistent and neuropathic pain. The Journal of Pharmacology and Experimental Therapeutics. 1996;**279**(3):1243-1249

[124] Mulroy MF, Greengrass R, Ganapathy S. Sameridine is safe and effective for spinal anesthesia: A comparative dose-ranging study with lidocaine for inguinal hernia repair. Anesthesia and Analgesia. 1999;**88**:815-821. DOI: 10.1097/00000539-199904000-00025

[125] Kafle S. Intrathecal meperidine for elective caesarean section: A comparison with lidocaine. Canadian Journal of Anaesthesia. 1993;**40**(8):718-721. DOI: 10.1007/BF03009767

[126] Strumper D, Durieux ME. Antidepressants as long-acting local anesthetics. Regional Anesthesia and Pain Medicine. 2004;**29**(3):277-285. DOI: 10.1016/j.rapm.2004.03.001

[127] De Araujo DR, Cereda CMS, Brunetto GB. Encapsulation of mepivacaine prolongs the analgesia provided by sciatic nerve blockade in mice. Canadian Journal of Anesthesia. 2004;**51**(6):566-572. DOI: 10.1007/BF03018399

[128] Boogaerts JG, Lafont ND, Declercq AG. Epidural administration of liposome associated bupivacaine for the management of postsurgical pain: A first study. Journal of Clinical Anesthesia. 1994;**6**(4):315-320. DOI: 10.1016/0952-8180(94)90079-5

[129] Gambling D, Hughes T, Martin G. A comparison of Depodur, a novel, single-dose extended-release epidural morphine, with standard epidural morphine for pain relief after lower abdominal surgery. Anesthesia and Analgesia. 2005;**100**(4):1065-1074. DOI: 10.1213/01.ANE.0000145009.03574.78

[130] Viscusi ER, Martin G, Hartrick CT. Forty-eight hours of postoperative pain relief after total hip arthroplasty with a novel, extended-release epidural morphine formulation. Anesthesiology. 2005;**102**(5):1014-1022. DOI: 10.1097/00000542-200505000-00022

[131] Carvalho B, Riley E, Cohen SE. Single-dose, sustained-release epidural morphine in the management of postoperative pain after elective cesarean delivery: Results of a multicenter randomized controlled study. Anesthesia and Analgesia. 2005;**100**(4):1150-1158. DOI: 10.1213/01.ANE.0000149544.58230.FF

[132] Grant SA. The holy grail: Long-acting local anaesthetics and liposomes. Best Practice & Research. Clinical Anaesthesiology. 2002;**16**(2):345-352. DOI: 10.1053/bean.2002.0242

Chapter 4

# Perspective Chapter: Epidural Administration – New Perspectives and Uses

*Allison Kalstein Apple, Sangeetha Kamath, Joel Yarmush, Sangeetha Setty, Vandana Gupta and Prabhdeep Singh*

## Abstract

Neuraxial techniques are commonplace in labor analgesia. Techniques for labor analgesia range from intrathecal and epidural anesthesia to peripheral nerve blocks, nitrous oxide, intravenous infusions, and acupuncture. The epidural approach is the most popular as it allows for local anesthetics to diffuse into the intrathecal space along with repeated or continuous doses of medication for labor and primary anesthetic for surgeries. The epidural technique affects differing spinal nerves (i.e., pain, autonomic, sensory, and motor) with varied effects depending on the concentration and volume of LA used. Adverse effects do exist following these techniques with hypotension being a major concern. A multitude of anesthetic agents can be given in the epidural; opioids are the most frequently used local anesthetic adjuvants. Alpha 2 adrenoreceptor agonists are also used as local anesthetic adjuvants. Although not performed routinely, peripheral nerve blocks play a complementary and supplementary role in epidural analgesia and anesthesia. There are absolute and relative contraindications to epidural anesthesia. Alternatives to neuraxial anesthesia that can be offered include infusion of ultrashort acting opioids, nitrous oxide, opioid agonist-antagonists, ketamine, TENS, and acupuncture. Local Anesthetic Systemic Toxicity may be more prevalent in the pregnant.

**Keywords:** neuraxial anesthesia, combined spinal epidural, intrathecal injection, local anesthetics, dural puncture technique, Accuro ultrasound, programmed intermittent epidural boluses, local anesthetic adjuvants, peripheral nerve blocks, LAST

## 1. Introduction

Spinal anesthesia is a neuraxial anesthesia technique in which local anesthetic (LA) is placed directly in the intrathecal (i.e., subarachnoid) space and blocks transmission of pain by the spinal nerves. The subarachnoid space houses sterile cerebrospinal fluid (CSF), the clear fluid that bathes the brain and spinal cord. Spinal anesthesia is only performed in the lumbar area, specifically the mid to low lumbar levels to avoid damage to the spinal cord and to prevent intrathecally injected medications from having any activity in the upper thoracic and cervical regions.

Epidural anesthesia is also a neuraxial technique. However, the LA is placed 'epi' or outside the intrathecal space. The LA (for the most part) then diffuses to the intrathecal space. This allows for potentially repeated doses via a catheter. It also can be placed in other regions (i.e., thoracic and cervical) of the neuraxis as well. The epidural thus has a larger breadth of applicability and can provide pain relief to a multitude of patients including those in labor, those for pain management, and those having a variety of surgeries.

New and exciting developments include ultrasound guidance to help with proper and more rapid placement of epidurals, newer equipment and devices to deliver medication in an improved manner, and recommended adjuvants to enhance the quality and the duration of the epidural. In addition to these developments, this chapter will explore adjunctive therapies such as regional blocks and acupuncture.

## 2. Outline

This chapter will cover basic anatomic considerations, basic general and obstetric physiology, basic epidural techniques and position, ultrasound use for epidural placement, pharmacological drugs used in epidurals, complimentary and supplementary regional blocks with epidurals, other remedies when epidurals are not viable or fail, and local anesthesia systemic toxicity (LAST).

## 3. Anatomy

From innermost to outermost layers, going toward the skin posteriorly, the spinal cord is surrounded by pia, arachnoid, and dura mater (see **Figure 1**) [1]. The epidural space is next, but it is only a potential fat-filled space that is formed between the dura mater of the spinal cord and the ligamentum flavum of the posterior vertebral column (see **Figure 2**). The posterior vertebral column is made up of bone (vertebrae) and the intervertebral space that has the ligamentum flavum, the interspinous ligament, and, finally, the supraspinous ligament. The vertebral pedicles and intervertebral foramina form the lateral limits of the epidural space. Longitudinally, the epidural space extends from the foramen magnum to the sacral hiatus. The vertebral column consists of 7 cervical, 12 thoracic, and 5 lumbar vertebrae and the corresponding intervertebral spaces and the sacrum and coccyx.

In adults, the spinal cord terminates at the level of the 1st and 2nd lumbar (L1–L2) vertebrae (see **Figure 3**) and is tethered to the coccyx. The spinal cord originates at L3, but after 1 year of age, the spinal cord moves upward (still tethered to the coccyx), creating a dural sac with CSF ending at the 2nd sacral vertebrae (S2) with many spinal nerves called the cauda equina. For safety, the epidural is placed below the L1–L2 vertebral interspace and above the sacrum that has no interspaces. The top of the iliac crest conveniently correlates with the L4–L5 interspace, and the L3–L4 or L4–L5 are the most common levels for insertion of the epidural. Problems with insertion include patients having scoliosis, osteophytes, calcifications, and diminished disc space because of vertebral fractures, to name a few.

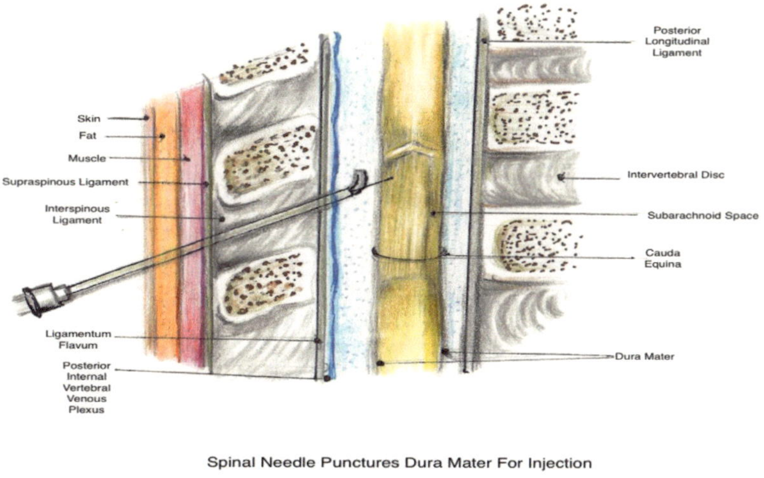


**Figure 1.**
*Spinal needle punctures dura mater for injection.*

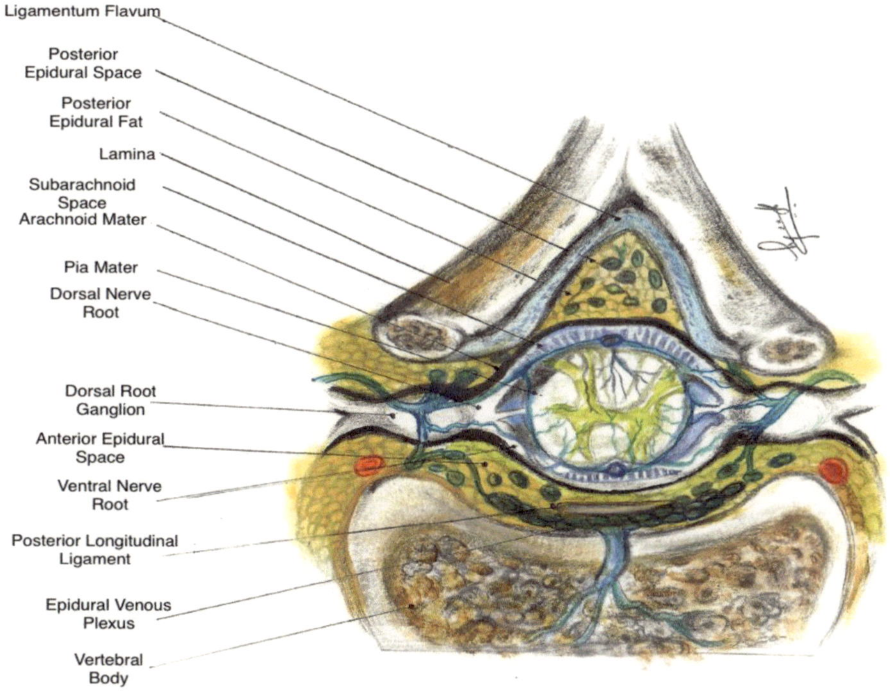


**Figure 2.**
*Cross section view of vertebral body.*

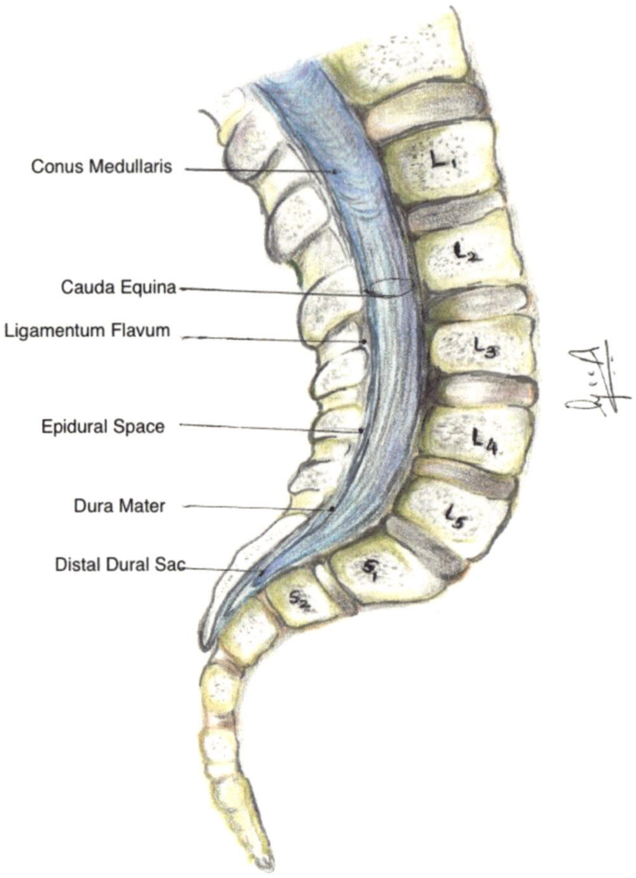


**Figure 3.**
*Side view of lumbosacral spine.*

## 4. Physiology

The epidural technique involves numbing different spinal nerves (i.e., pain, autonomic, sensory, and motor) with varied effects depending on the concentration and volume of LA used. Regardless of which nerves are blocked, there is a physiologic consequence to blocking these nerves. In particular, hypotension is the major potential problem due to blocking the sensitive sympathetic fibers and causing vasodilation [2, 3]. This hypotension, if severe enough, may lead to decreased organ perfusion and in the extreme organ dysfunction.

Another problem is the level of spread of LA. If the spread is too high (i.e., rostral), the intercostal muscles may be blocked, leading to an uncomfortable feeling of not being able to take a deep breath. If the spread is too low (i.e., caudal), the urinary muscles may be blocked leading to difficulty in urinating. Thus, targeting the right level is important. This is especially so in the parturient population.

Parturients in labor are the largest group of patients receiving an epidural. Knowing the stages of labor gives more insight into the level of epidural analgesia required. The first stage of labor includes cervical dilation and uterine contractions. The neural signaling via the sympathetic chain will enter the spinal cord at T10 –L1

(**Figure 4**), causing visceral pain to the parturient. If the epidural is placed at the L3–L4 or L4–L5 interspace, a bolus of 10–15 ml of LA would be necessary to affect the appropriate level.

In the second stage of labor, the fetal head descends, and the pain becomes more somatic in nature, with vaginal and perineal stretching as the pain is transmitted through the pudendal nerves at S2–S4 (see **Figure 4**). If the epidural is placed at the L3–L4 or L4–L5 interspace, a bolus of 20–25 ml of LA would be necessary to affect the appropriate level.

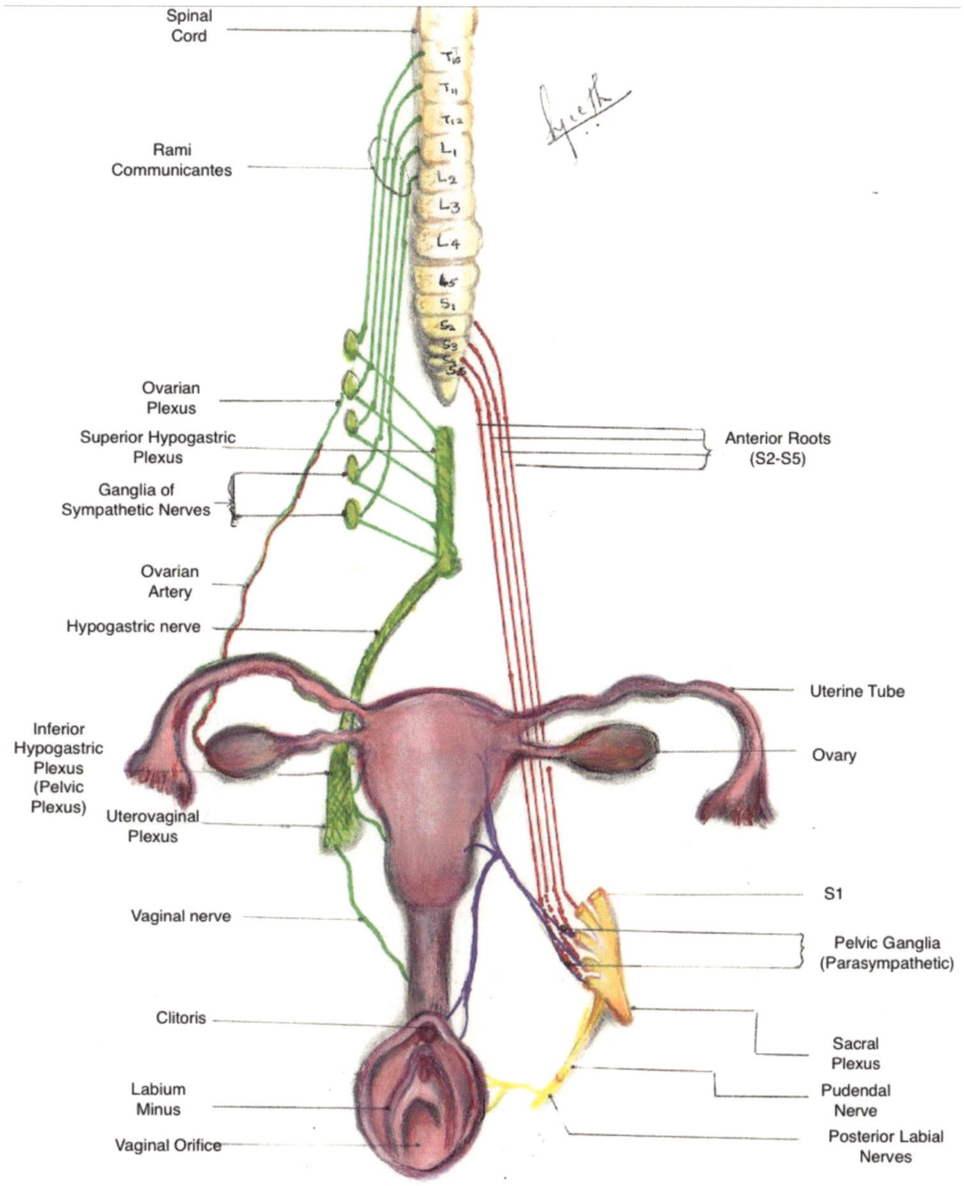


**Figure 4.**
*Sensory innervation from lumbosacral plexus.*

## 5. Epidural techniques and position

As stated in the introduction, the epidural is used because a catheter can be placed in the epidural space, allowing redosing. There are at least two alternatives to the classic epidural. One involves the placement of an epidural catheter combined with a spinal block and is called a combined spinal epidural (CSE). The intrathecal dose is administered before the catheter is placed. In the other, an epidural catheter is again placed after a spinal puncture, but no actual intrathecal dose is given, and this is called a dural puncture technique (DPT).

The classic epidural involves the placement of a catheter in the epidural space, a bolus dose of medication, and continuous medication infused into the epidural space through a pump. The bolus dose may take a bit of time to work as it has to diffuse into the intrathecal space.

The CSE offers a quicker onset of pain relief with the continued advantage of analgesia from the epidural infusion. In addition, confirming the CSF through the spinal needle allows the provider to feel confident that he or she is in the correct spot when placing the epidural. This confirms that the loss of resistance is not false (discussed later). While there is a small chance of post dural puncture headache (PDPH) with the dural puncture, the use of a very small gauge needle for the spinal puncture will decrease the chance to almost negligible. The quicker onset of the CSE may lead to unwanted hypotension, though. This hypotension can be mitigated by adding fluids and the use of vasopressors like phenylephrine and ephedrine.

The DPT is a compromise between the classic epidural and the CSE and is quicker than the classic epidural but has less hypotension than the CSE.

Most practitioners find it easier to place the epidural in the sitting position. The patient's midline can be easily determined in the sitting position. There are five layers that a practitioner must pass through from a midline position in order to get to the epidural space (see **Figure 1**). These layers are the skin, the subcutaneous fat, the supraspinous ligament, the interspinous ligament, and the ligamentum flavum. While sitting, spinal flexion and neutral rotation should be achieved to establish a straight path for needle insertion in the intervertebral space between the spinous processes. It is helpful to first feel the landmarks, which include the top of the iliac crests correlating to the L4–L5 interspace. Additionally, it helps to feel the spinous processes and trace them down from cervical to thoracic to lumbar to identify if the patient has any scoliosis or curvature, which may make the procedure more difficult. Once the interspace is identified, one can place a mark at the chosen location. It is important to clean the back well in a sterile fashion. Chlorhexidine has been found to be superior to betadine in recent studies and is recommended unless the patient has an allergy to chlorhexidine. Typically, chlorhexidine should be allowed to dry for at least three minutes. Next, the epidural kit should be set up while allowing the chlorhexidine to dry. The procedure starts with injecting LA liberally with a 3/8 inch 25-gauge needle in the skin and subcutaneous space to numb the area. A longer (i.e., 1 ½ inch) 25-gauge finder needle may be used to determine the location of the interspace past the subcutaneous tissue. The epidural needle, usually a 17-gauge blunt Tuohy needle with obturator in place, is advanced in the same plane as the finder needle and is seated in the interspinous ligament. The obturator is removed, and a glass saline-filled syringe is attached to the Tuohy needle, and the resistance of the ligament is felt, preventing any saline from being injected. The Tuohy needle–glass syringe assembly is advanced very slowly, feeling for resistance every 1–2 mm. When the ligamentum flavum is reached, there may be, but often not, a subtle change in resistance. After

*DOI: http://dx.doi.org/10.5772/intechopen.109691*

passing the ligamentum flavum, there is a sudden loss of resistance, and the saline can be easily injected.

After the loss of resistance is confirmed, the glass syringe is removed carefully, and an epidural catheter is threaded into the epidural space through the Tuohy needle. The epidural catheter is placed 4–6 cm beyond the Tuohy needle into the epidural space. After catheter placement, the Tuohy needle is removed with careful attention as to not remove the newly placed catheter.

There may be problems placing the epidural catheter. A false loss of resistance may be obtained if the resistance of the ligament is not very obvious because of patient characteristics and so on. The patient may have an altered or difficult anatomy preventing the midline approach. When a midline approach is difficult, a paramedian approach can be tried. In the paramedian approach, the needle should be inserted 1–2 cm lateral to the inferior tip of the posterior spinous process, corresponding to the vertebra above the desired interspace. The needle is then advanced horizontally until the lamina is reached and then redirected medially and cephalad to enter the epidural space [4].

While an intrathecal puncture with a very small gauge needle will usually not cause a PDPH, an intrathecal puncture with the large 17-gauge bore Tuohy needle will almost certainly cause a PDPH, which may result in exaggerated complications. An ultrasound device may be helpful in preventing this occurrence.

## 6. Use of ultrasound

The ultrasound is a helpful tool, as one can have direct vision while placing the epidural, or at least visualize the midline when it is not visible secondary to calcifications, spina bifida, or instrumentation. In cases of obese patients or patients with scoliosis, the ultrasound can be particularly useful.

Using the ultrasound, a practitioner may see the midline and the depth at which the loss of resistance should occur. This lessens the risks of false loss of resistance and incorrect placement in the obese patients and fewer unwanted dural punctures with the Tuohy needle and less chance of headache in the ultrathin patients. The ultrasound is a radiation-free technique and therefore may be safely used in the obstetric patients. In addition, Rivanna produces the Accuro, which is a handheld, portable ultrasound. The Accuro uses 3D as well as 2D technology to line up the intralaminar and the epidural space. The device allows for the depth of the epidural space to be noted, allowing easier epidural placement.

## 7. Medications

A multitude of anesthetic agents can be given in the epidural to provide analgesia or anesthesia for procedures or surgeries. LAs work by inhibiting conduction of nerve impulses, by binding to a subunit of the voltage-gated sodium channels and impairing nerve impulses. When the sodium ions are prevented from entering the cell, the nerve conduction is inhibited.

LAs are classified as either amides or esters [5]. Amides are more stable in solutions, whereas esters are less stable. The amino esters are hydrolyzed by pseudocholinesterase in plasma, while amides undergo enzymatic degradation by the liver and are excreted in the urine. Common amide Las include lidocaine, bupivacaine, and ropivacaine. Common ester anesthetics include procaine, chloropropane, and tetracaine. Esters generally cause a greater degree of allergic reactions, due to the metabolites of amino esters, like para-aminobenzoic acid, which can cause an immunological response.

LAs block different nerves depending on the concentration of the LAs and the size (i.e., sensitivity) of the nerve. The smallest nerves that are the most sensitive are the pain, temperature, and autonomic nerves. The medium nerves that are less sensitive are the sensory nerves. The large nerves that are fairly resistant are the motor nerves, and the largest and most resistant are the positional nerves. Epidural analgesia for labor usually requires a more dilute LA solution, while epidural anesthesia for cesarean section requires a more concentrated LA solution.

Lidocaine is the archetypical LA. At a concentration of 0.5%, a bolus of lidocaine will block transmission to the pain, temperature, and autonomic fibers. At a concentration of 1.0%, a bolus of lidocaine will block sensory fibers. At a concentration of 2.0%, a bolus of lidocaine will block motor fibers. However, there is an overlap, and at 0.5%, the bolus may affect some sensory fibers, and at 1%, the bolus may affect some motor fibers. An infusion of LA requires a lesser concentration for the same effect on the nerves and may be given continuously. An infusion of 0.25, 0.5, and 1% lidocaine will block the smaller, medium, and large nerves, respectively.

Lidocaine is of medium onset and lasts a medium duration of time. Bupivacaine is of slower onset but lasts much longer, while chloroprocaine is of fast onset but lasts a short time. 0.125, 0.25, and 0.5% bupivacaine boluses and 1, 2, and 3% chloroprocaine boluses correspond to lidocaine boluses. A 0.0625, 0.125, and 0.25% bupivacaine infusion and a 0.5, 1, and 2% chloroprocaine infusion correspond to a lidocaine infusion. Ropivacaine and levobupivacaine are the only commercially available single-enantiomer local anesthetics, these were initially developed as less cardiotoxic alternatives to bupivacaine [6].

The concentration and volume of LAs determine LAST (discussed later). A lesser concentration and hence safer mixture of LAs may be used if other drugs (namely, adjuvants) are added to the mix. Some adjuvants (i.e., bicarbonate) decrease the onset time; some adjuvants (i.e., epinephrine) prolong the duration of block; some adjuvants (i.e., opioids) enhance the analgesia.

By adding these adjuvants, it is possible to give such a dilute mixture of LAs that will allow the patient to ambulate and be pain-free with few side effects. This is known as a 'walking' epidural. There are many combinations of these mixtures. One such combination is ropivacaine 0.025% with fentanyl 3 mcg/ml and epinephrine 0.5 mcg/ml [7].

Also, not all infusions are the same. Rather than using the traditional continuous infusion techniques for labor, the new programmed intermittent epidural boluses (PIEBs) are thought to provide better analgesia and lower anesthesia requirements overall. The PIEB allows for the patient to get a spray of epidural medications, covering more dermatomes and adding to analgesic satisfaction and less motor block. Unlike the traditional continuous epidural infusions that deposit medication in the same location, the PIEB allows the epidural infusion to be spread over a greater area [8]. PIEB labor analgesia has a higher threshold for motor blockade because the intraneural concentration is reduced as local anesthetic diffuses out of the nerve between boluses.

Properties: Local anesthetics that have an increased lipid solubility are associated with enhanced diffusion through neuronal coverings and lower milligram dosage and hence higher potency. In contrast, those local anesthetics which are lipid-insoluble are more highly protein bound in the blood and have a longer duration [9]. The baricity of a local anesthesia is used to determine where the local anesthetic will spread in the intrathecal space. Dissociation constant determines the portion of the drug that stays in the lipid soluble tertiary molecular state (lower PKa) and hastens onset.

Opioids are the most frequently used local anesthetic adjuvants, and their use in neuraxial blocks has evolved over the last 50 years. The dose, site of injection, lipophilicity, and the acid-base milieu of the site of drug deposition determine the extent of efficacy of the block. They can be given intrathecally or epidurally. Typically, the epidural dose is 5–10 times the intrathecal dose as the epidurally placed drug must diffuse to the intrathecal space to work. The opioids used as adjuvants have differing properties. Morphine must be prepared as a preservative-free solution. The hydrophilic nature of neuraxial morphine results in cephalad spread, thereby increasing the area and duration of analgesia. However, the adverse effect of its use in neuraxial blocks includes respiratory depression (early and late), nausea, vomiting, pruritus, and urinary retention. Fentanyl has been shown to have a lesser prolongation of block compared with neuraxial morphine with a more favorable adverse effect profile. The addition of epinephrine to the fentanyl results in a slightly further prolongation with still better adverse-effect profile, especially less nausea. The use of epinephrine 1:1000 or 1:10000 along with lidocaine and fentanyl in spinal anesthesia in women candidates for C-section produced no statistically significant difference in the hemodynamic, post-operative nausea and vomiting and post-operative paralysis and pain relief [10, 11].

Epinephrine is a potent vasoconstrictor that decreases absorption into the vasculature. This results in an increase of duration of block and an increase in the systemic safety profile. It by itself may also add some analgesia.

Adding epinephrine to an LA with or without opioids allows for a more dilute LA solution, and in the extreme, the dilute concentration of an LA together with a dilute concentration of opioid allows a parturient to have pain relief (especially during the first stage of labor) with virtually no effect on the motor nerves. A 'walking' epidural can be sometimes be achieved with a solution of 0.0625% bupivacaine 2 mcg/ml of fentanyl and 5 mcg/ml of epinephrine.

Alpha 2 adrenoreceptor agonists (Clonidine, Dexmedetomidine) are also used as local anesthetic adjuvants. They act on postjunctional alpha-2 adrenoreceptor in the dorsal horn of spinal cord.

Neuraxially, they have a local effect on the blockage of sympathetic outflow, while peripherally, they prolong the duration of analgesia by hyperpolarization of cation channels [12]. Epidural clonidine in doses of 25–50 mcg/h has been found to have fewer side effects. Intrathecal administration of clonidine has evolved in terms of dosing from the initial phases of higher doses (i.e., 150 mcg) to routine use of lesser doses (i.e., 15–40 mcg) in present-day practice to avoid its cardiovascular adverse effects.

Dexmedetomidine is a 7-times more selective alpha-2 receptor agonist in comparison to clonidine and has a similar mechanism of blocking hyperpolarization activated cation channels. Intrathecal (5–10 mcg) and epidural dexmedetomidine (1 mcg/kg) as an adjuvant to isobaric bupivacaine or in combination with the commonly used LA has been investigated for its analgesic efficacy in various patient subsets. Its use has been associated with prolonged duration of block and improved postoperative analgesia without any associated hypotension or other adverse events, especially when used at doses less than 5 mcg. However, it is often associated with a higher incidence of bradycardia. Comparative evaluation of dexmedetomidine and clonidine has revealed the superiority of dexmedetomidine when used as an adjuvant for epidural or intrathecal administration.

Dexamethasone is a potent steroidal anti-inflammatory agent and can be used as an adjuvant. There is evidence to suggest that dexamethasone has analgesic properties in addition to increasing the duration of LA action.

## 8. Peripheral nerve blocks

Although not performed routinely, peripheral nerve blocks (PNBs) play a complementary and supplementary role in epidural analgesia and anesthesia.

The lumbar paravertebral block (PVB) is placed outside the dura mater by the paraspinal space and is used when a standard epidural is not or cannot be used. The typical dermatomal spread for a single-level block with an injected volume of 5 mL is four dermatomal levels. A bilateral PVB at the T12–L1 level is used for a cesarean section. In addition, visceral pain can be treated with a paravertebral sympathetic block (PSB) that prevents pain from uterine innervation via the preganglionic and postganglionic sympathetic fibers of the superior and inferior hypogastric plexus (branches of the hypogastric nerve).

The major advantage of paravertebral nerve blocks is that analgesia can be provided in patients for whom neuraxial analgesia could be complicated, such as neuraxial anatomical abnormalities or spine surgery with instrumentation. The duration of analgesia with typical agents is 9–12 h.

The transversus abdominis plane (TAP) block is a field block of the thoracolumbar nerves that run in the fascial plane between the internal oblique muscle and the transversus abdominis muscles (**Figure 5**), the anterior primary rami course between the internal oblique and the transversus abdominis muscles, and, subsequently, branch into the lateral and anterior cutaneous nerves at approximately the midaxillary line. It is used to complement a neuraxial block. The major disadvantage is that it does not provide visceral analgesia. This omission explains why many studies have failed

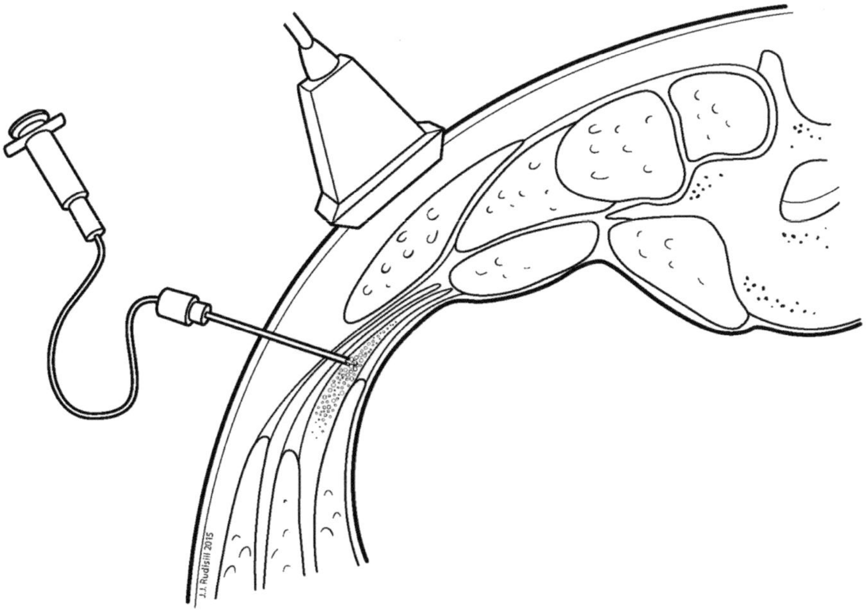


**Figure 5.**
*Illustration of transversus abdominis plane (TAP) block.*

to show the superiority of TAP or give mixed results when compared with standard multimodal analgesia.

The quadratus lumborum block (QLB) is also a field block of the thoracolumbar nerves but is placed more laterally (**Figure 6**). Its posterior spread into the paravertebral space can potentially affect the sympathetic chain, conferring some visceral as well as somatic analgesia. The QLB seems to have a greater dermatomal spread than the TAP block.

The disadvantage of the block is that it is more difficult than a TAP block, and it has greater systemic absorption through the highly vascularized muscle bed, potentially causing local systemic anesthetic toxicity.

An erector spinae plane block (ESPB) involves truncal deposition of LA in the plane anterior to the erector spinae muscles and superficial to the transverse processes of thoracic or lumbar vertebrae, resulting in considerable spread in both cephalo-caudad and medial-lateral directions. This is a complementary block for neuraxial anesthesia after cesarean section.

The disadvantage of this block is that it is difficult to place.

A paracervical block is a supplementary block for the first stage of labor when a neuraxial block is inadequate. It can be placed by the obstetric team especially if a neuraxial block team is unavailable (**Figure 7**).

The disadvantage of the paracervical block is that it has a high incidence of fetal bradycardia, and it does not help with the second stage of labor.

A pudendal nerve block is a supplementary block for the second stage of labor when a neuraxial block is inadequate. It too can be placed by the obstetric team especially if a neuraxial block team is unavailable.

The disadvantage of the pudendal block is that it alone does not provide reliable analgesia for the second stage of labor as both the cervical and pudendal nerves must be blocked. However, the block is useful for episiotomy and repair (**Figure 8**).

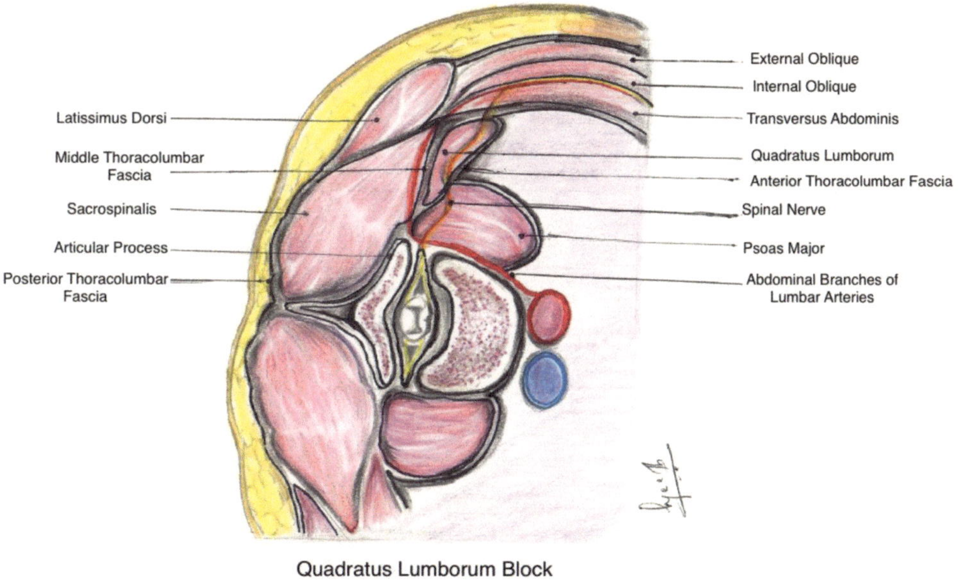


**Figure 6.**
*Quadratus lumborum block.*

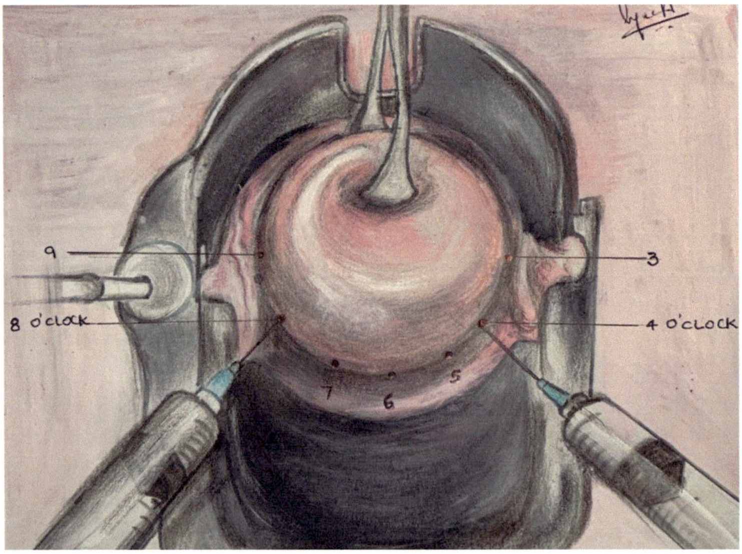


**Figure 7.**
*Illustration of paracervical block.*

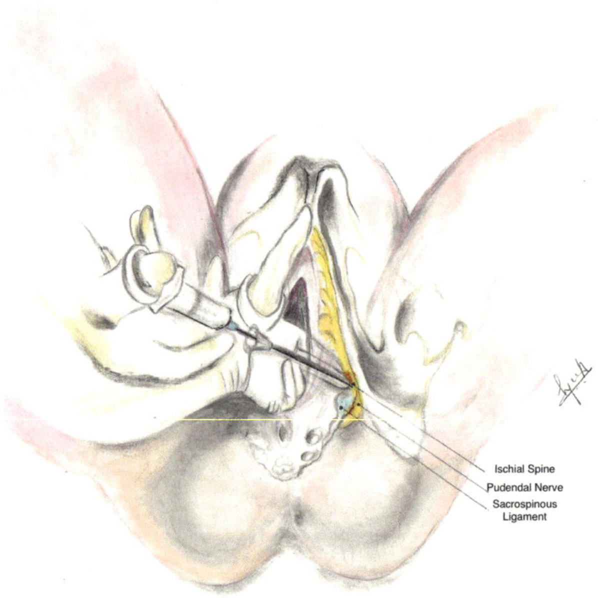


**Figure 8.**
*Illustration of pudendal nerve block.*

Liposomal bupivacaine may also be used for the peripheral nerve blocks. Liposomal bupivacaine is a prolonged-release (up to 72 h) formulation of bupivacaine approved by the US Federal Drug Administration for postoperative analgesia by single-dose infiltration. It is expensive to use, and not many centers approve its use (**Figure 9**).

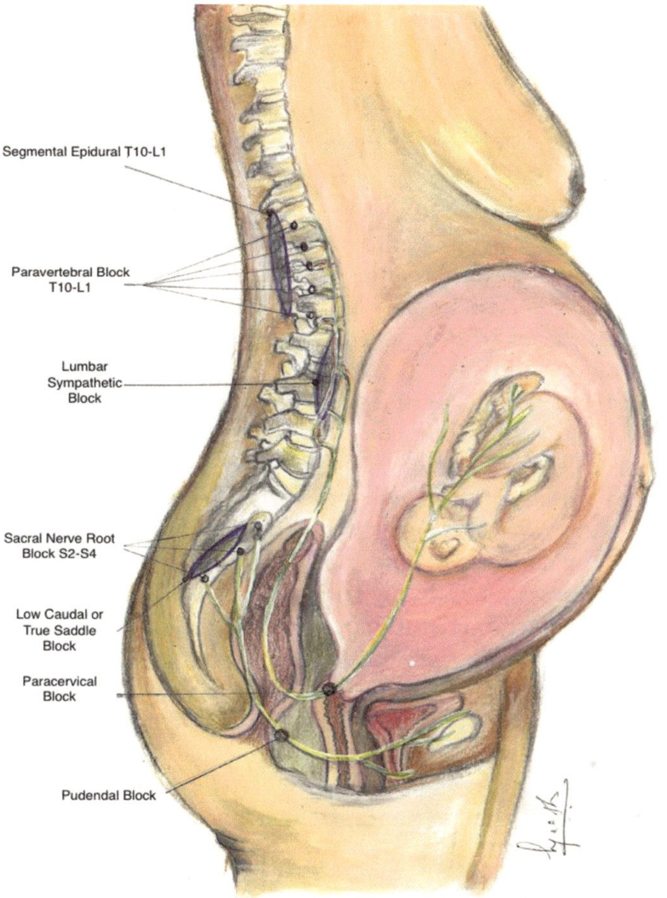


**Figure 9.**
*Different block levels for labor analgesia.*

## 9. When you need something besides an epidural

There are both absolute and relative contraindications to epidural anesthesia. The absolute contraindications include patient refusal, localized sepsis in the area where the neuraxial anesthesia is to be performed, an allergy to the medications used [13, 14], and severe coagulopathy such as disseminated intravascular coagulation.

Thrombocytopenia has previously been considered a contraindication for neuraxial anesthesia; however, recently, the consensus regarding platelets has been changing. Rather than looking at an absolute number, the overall platelet trend can help to determine if a patient is a good candidate for neuraxial anesthesia. In 2016, the ASA practice guidelines for obstetric anesthesia stated that it is unnecessary to have a routine platelet count for a healthy parturient [9]. Coagulation profile is also not recommended unless the parturient has a history of coagulopathy, preeclampsia, or HELLP syndrome. While there is no minimum platelet count, 70,000 platelet count has been an acceptable number [15, 16].

Relative contraindications include generalized fever or infection, spina bifida, multiple sclerosis, anticoagulation, central nervous system disorders and preload dependent states (i.e., aortic stenosis), previous back surgery or instrumentation, placement in anesthetized adults, and needle placement through a tattoo [17].

An ultrashort acting opioid such as remifentanil may be used. Remifentanil is rapidly metabolized by serum and tissue cholinesterases and consequently has an acceptable level of maternal side effects with minimal or no fetal side effects.

Nitrous oxide (N2O) may also be used especially in countries where neuraxial analgesia is unavailable. Remifentanil may offer better pain relief than nitrous oxide with fewer side effects. However, N2O can still be used.

N2O is a nonflammable, tasteless, and odorless gas. N2O is always delivered with oxygen in a 50:50 mixture. It can be used for the first and second stages of labor as well as during postdelivery procedures such as laceration repair, manual removal of the placenta, and uterine curettage. It may also facilitate the initiation of epidural analgesia. N2O is self-administered and has a rapid onset of 30 to 50 seconds. N2O administration is intermittent and delivered via face mask. The patient's inhalation triggers the opening of a negative pressure demand valve and is timed by the patient to coincide with uterine contractions. Anecdotal reports have noted the patient report of greatest relief when the woman begins inhalation approximately 30 seconds prior to the start of her contraction. This pattern of inhalation allows for peak serum levels of N2O to coincide with the peak of the uterine contraction. Offset is rapid, with elimination of the N2O by exhalation occurring within a few minutes of discontinuation. It is important that the N2O be administered by the patient herself using a handheld face mask; no straps or other devices should be used to secure the mask to the patient's face that could lead to excessive drowsiness. Learning the correct technique by practicing with the first few contractions is important in order to maximize results. Patient satisfaction and success with therapy can be enhanced by thorough teaching with a focus on the timing of breathing. Pain relief is less effective than with neuraxial analgesia utilizing local anesthetics.

Environmental pollution can occur with the use of N2O, and a scavenger system is required. Increased access to N2O services in hospitals and birth centers has long been advocated by the midwifery profession. A position statement on Nitrous Oxide for Labor Analgesia issued by the American College of Nurse-Midwives in 2009 advocates for the availability of N2O to all laboring women and recommends that all certified nurse-midwives and certified midwives be trained "to administer and oversee safe use of N2O analgesia during labor" [18]. The American Society of Anesthesiology and the American Congress of Obstetricians and Gynecologists do not currently have any position statements regarding N2O use for labor analgesia.

Inability to obtain CSF, sometimes referred to as a 'dry tap', is one of the causes of failure of the intrathecal portion of a CSE or DPT. A failed lumbar puncture is usually because of poor positioning of the patient or incorrect needle insertion, both factors being within the control of the anesthetist. Abnormalities of the spine (kyphosis, scoliosis, calcification of ligaments, and consequences of osteoporosis), obesity, and patient anxiety make both positioning the patient and needle insertion more difficult. The appearance of clear fluid at the needle hub is usually the final confirmation that the subarachnoid space has been entered. Intrathecal spread is governed by the interplay between solution, physical characteristics, gravity, and the configuration of the vertebral canal. Anatomical abnormalities can lead to problems with spread. The curves of the vertebral column are integral to solution spread, and any obvious abnormality, kyphosis, or scoliosis may interfere with the process. The epidural should hopefully still work, but analgesia may be delayed.

Systemic medications may also be used if the epidural is inconvenient or has failed. Opioid agonist-antagonists, such as butorphanol and nalbuphine, have also been used for obstetric analgesia when an epidural is inconvenient or has failed. These analgesic drugs may have a lower incidence of nausea and vomiting [19]. Butorphanol is probably the most popular of the mixed agonist-antagonists. A disadvantage is a high incidence of maternal sedation. The recommended dose is 1–2 mg by IV or IM injection.

Nalbuphine 10 mg IV or IM is an alternative to butorphanol.

Ketamine is another analgesic drug that is often used specifically if the epidural is 'patchy' or incomplete. In low doses (0.2–0.4 mg/kg), ketamine provides analgesia without causing neonatal depression. However, ketamine has sedative and amnestic properties that may be troublesome for the parturient.

Alternate techniques such as TENS and acupuncture in labor have been tried, but the results are at best mixed. One controlled study comparing acupuncture to no treatment for labor pain concluded that acupuncture was not effective, but a non-controlled study (i.e., without a comparator) on a larger population concluded that acupuncture was effective [20]. Acupuncture has been shown to be helpful in alleviating anxiety even in laboring patients.

## 10. Local Anesthetic Systemic Toxicity (LAST)

For obstetric patients, LAST may be more prevalent than the nonpregnant population secondary to decreased protein binding, increased tissue blood flow, and vascular engorgement. Data suggest that up to 20 out of 10,000 peripheral nerve blocks and 4 out of 10,000 epidural blocks result in systemic local anesthetic toxicity [21].

The systemic toxicity initially manifests as central nervous system toxicity. The patient may feel lightheaded, dizzy, have ringing in the ears, and trouble focusing. As the systemic toxicity progresses, excitatory symptoms such as shivering, tremors, muscle twitching, and even seizures appear, resulting from an initial blockade of inhibitory pathways by the local anesthetic drugs [17]. As the toxicity progresses further, cardiac manifestations appear. This may result in severe hypotension, atrioventricular conduction delay, idioventricular rhythms, and, eventually, cardiovascular collapse [7].

Local anesthetic toxicity is difficult to treat, and lipid containing solutions to absorb the local anesthetic are used. In particular, Intralipid, a 20% fat emulsion, is used.

Also, the seizure threshold can be raised by giving a small dose of benzodiazepine such as midazolam, if CNS toxicity is suspected.

## Author details

Allison Kalstein Apple*, Sangeetha Kamath, Joel Yarmush, Sangeetha Setty, Vandana Gupta and Prabhdeep Singh
Affiliates of New York Presbyterian Brooklyn Methodist Hospital, New York, USA

*Address all correspondence to: ka2600@hotmail.com

## References

[1] Miller RD, Cohen NH, Eriksson LI, Fleisher LA, Wiener-Kronish JP, Young W. Miller's Anesthesia. 8th ed. Vol. 1. Philadelphia, PA: Elsevier; 2015. pp. 1685-1686

[2] Veering BT, Cousins MJ. Cardiovascular and pulmonary effects of epidural anesthesia. Anaesthesia and Intensive Care. 2000;**28**(6):620-635. DOI: 10.1177/0310057X0002800603

[3] Liu MD, Randall L, Neal JM. Epidural anesthesia and analgesia: Their role in postoperative outcome spencer. Anesthesiology. 1995;**82**:1474-1506. DOI:10.1097/00000542-199506000-00019

[4] Miller R, Cohen N, Eriksson L, Fleisher L, Wiener-Kronish J, Young WL. Miller's Anesthesia. 8th ed. Vol. 1. Philadelphia, PA: Elsevier; 2015. p. 1709

[5] Barash PG, Cullen BF, Stoelting RK, Cahalan MK, Stock MC, Ortega R, et al. Clinical Anesthesiology. 8th ed. Philadelphia, PA: Wolters. pp. 569-933

[6] Barash PG, Cullen BF, Stoelting RK, Cahalan MK, Stock MC, Ortega R, et al. Clinical Anesthesiology. 8th ed. Philadelphia, PA: Wolters. pp. 568-570

[7] Cohen S, Chhokra R, Stein MH, Denny JT, Shah S, Mohiuddin A, et al. Ropivacaine 0.025% mixed with fentanyl 3.0 μg/ml and epinephrine 0.5 μg/ml is effective for epidural patient-controlled analgesia after cesarean section. Journal of Anaesthesiology and Clinical Pharmacology. 2015;**31**(4):471-477. DOI: 10.4103/0970-9185.169065

[8] Mo X, Zhao T, Chen J, Li X, Liu J, Xu C, et al. Programmed intermittent epidural bolus in comparison with continuous epidural infusion for uterine contraction pain relief after cesarean section: A Randomized, Double-Blind Clinical Trial. 2022;**2022**:999-1009

[9] Butterworth J. "Clinical Pharmacology of Local Anesthetics." NYSORA. 8 Jun 2018. Available from: www.nysora.com/topics/pharmacology/clinical-pharmacology-local-anesthetics/#toc_REFERENCES. [Accessed: 07 Dec 2022]

[10] Chamberlain BK, Volpe P, Fleischer S. Inhibition of calcium-induced calcium release from purified cardiac sarcoplasmic reticulum vesicles. Journal of Biological Chemistry. 25 Jun 1984;**259**(12):7547-7553. PMID: 6736019

[11] Hamzei A, Nazemi SH, Alami A, Gochan DMA, Kazemi A. Comparing Different Epinephrine Concentrations for Spinal Anesthesia in Cesarean Section: A Double-Blind Randomized Clinical Trial. Iran Journal of Medical Sciences Research. Jul 2015;**40**(4):302-308. PMID: 26170515; PMCID: PMC4487454

[12] Ok S-H, Hong J-M, Sohn J-T. Lipid emulsion for treating local anesthetic systemic toxicity. International Journal of Medical Sciences. 14 May 2018;**15**(7):713-722. DOI: 10.7150/ijms.22643. PMID: 29910676; PMCID: PMC6001420

[13] Stiles P, Prielipp R. Intralipid treatment of bupicavaine toxicity. Anesthesia Patient Safety Foundation, Circulation. Volume 24, No. 1, Spring 2009

[14] Choi J, Germond L, Santos AC. Obstetric Regional Anesthesia. NYSORA. 5 Jul 2018. Available from: www.nysora.com/topics/sub-specialties/obstetric/obstetric-regional-anesthesia/ [Accessed: 07 Dec 2022]

[15] Adjuvants to local anesthetics: Current understanding and future

trends. World Journal of Clinical Cases. 2017;**5**(8):307-323. DOI: 10.12998/wjcc.v5.i8.307

[16] Lyrenas S, et al. Acupuncture before delivery: Effect on pain perception and the need for analgesics. Gynecology Obstetrics Investigations. 1990;**29**:188-224

[17] A review of peripheral nerve blocks for cesarean delivery analgesia. Regional Anesthesia Pain and Medicine. 2021. DOI: 10.1136/rapm-2019-100752

[18] Collins MR, Starr SA, Bishop JT, Baysinger CL. Nitrous oxide for labor analgesia: expanding analgesic options for women in the United States. Rev Obstet Gynecol. 2012;**5**(3-4):e126-e131. PMID: 23483795; PMCID: PMC3594866

[19] Fettes PDW, Jansson J-R, Wildsmith JAW. Failed spinal anesthesia: Mechanisms, management, and prevention. BJA: British Journal of Anesthesia. 2009;**102**(6):739-748. DOI: 10.1093/bja/aep096

[20] Martoudis S, Christofides K. Electroacupuncture for pain relief in labor. Acupuncture in Medicine. 1990;**8**:51-53

[21] Practice Guidelines for Obstetric Anesthesia. An updated report by the American Society of Anesthesiologists Task Force on Obstetric Anesthesia and the Society for Obstetric Anesthesia and Perinatology. Anesthesiology. 2016;**124**:270-300. DOI: 10.1097/ALN.0000000000000935

Section 3

# Epidural Administration and Cell-Based Therapy

Chapter 5

# Perspectives of Cell-Based Therapy for Degenerative Diseases of the Spine: The Reason for Choosing the Epidural Space

*José Correa, Henry Cortés, Lucia Correa and Rita López*


## Abstract

Intervertebral disc degeneration (IDD) is a chronic disease that causes significant disability and dependence and exerts a high cost on society. Concerning IDD, it is the most common cause of back pain, involving any segment of the spine. It is one of the most frequent reasons for consultation in the general population, second only to headache, affecting 80–85 % of people throughout life. Current therapeutic strategies focused on IDD are primarily conservative, including physical therapy and antiinflammatory medication. Surgical techniques intend to stabilize the spine and/or decompress the spinal or foraminal canal, searching for relieve of symptoms; however, do not address the cause of the degeneration and even accelerate the degeneration of adjacent segments. Understanding of the biology of platelet-rich plasma (PRP) and other growth factors conducted usto use of PRP as a promising biological therapeutic strategy for enhance the regenerative process, searching the healing of the intervertebral disc. With current few in vitro studies, and fewer clinical studies linking the bases of regenerative medicine (RM) in the management of degenerative disc disease, our pioneering research was to state the bases, fundamentals, results, and the new trends around the RM techniques focused on the pathology of the spinal canal, taking the advantages that offer the epidural route.


**Keywords:** epidural space, intervertebral disc degeneration, intervertebral disc regeneration, platelet-rich plasma, tissue engineering

## 1. Introduction

Low back pain (LBP) has become a major public health issue for people under 45 years. This global problem has an estimated prevalence of about 7.5% in the global population (WHO, 2017). LBP is a costly and challenging condition to manage. LBP has become one of the main reasons for limiting of physical activities and is spreading in epidemic proportions [1, 2]. With these concerns in mind, it is important to highlight that lumbar disc degeneration is the most common cause of low back pain. Intervertebral disc disease (IDD) is a progressive, chronic disorder and number one cause of LBP.

Understanding of the IDD pathophysiology and its clinical course will allow us to focus on a rational treatment for the patient, when possible. Current treatments for IDD proposed in most´ consensus protocols´ do not correspond, unfortunately, to the pathophysiological process involved in the IDD, as these treatments are mainly focused on relieving pain (palliative pain medicine) [3]. Recent studies addressing the treatment of LBP, as opposed to current protocols, focus their management strategy based on the genesis that triggers pain. These pioneering studies [4–6] show that epidural PRP injections can improve significantly in the pain score (VAS-scale) and function (MACNAB-score) in patients with IDD diagnosis.

The aim of this chapter is to overview our pioneering research, the bases, fundamentals, and results. Also, this research includes the near future around the regenerative medicine (RM) techniques associated to the medullary canal. This research document also aims to highlight the new trends what the Regenerative Medicine focuses on the pathology of the spinal canal.

## 2. Historical overview

### 2.1 The evolution from general anesthesia to spinal techniques

*... at past, surgeries were horrible ...*

The beginning of Anesthesia dates to ancient civilization, seeking to alter the consciousness to prevent pain during surgery. Deliriant herbs as the sleeping sponge (Hippocrates), opium, belladonna, scopolamine, cannabis were the herbal remedies as anesthetics (**Figure 1**). At the XVI century appeared ether (Paracelsus) through the distillation of alcohol and sulfuric acid. Already in 1796 Davy discovered nitrous oxide (N2O) opening the doors to the future of anesthesia [7].

The knowledge of the chemical agents that altered the consciousness, and later the control of mechanical ventilation, through pulmonary insufflation, allowed the use of other drugs, no longer focused to pain control, but to facilitate the conditions of surgery. Appeared then the use of muscle relaxants and other drugs that allowed the control of the hemodynamic conditions of the patient. It came up the concept safety during surgery, the beginning of monitoring.

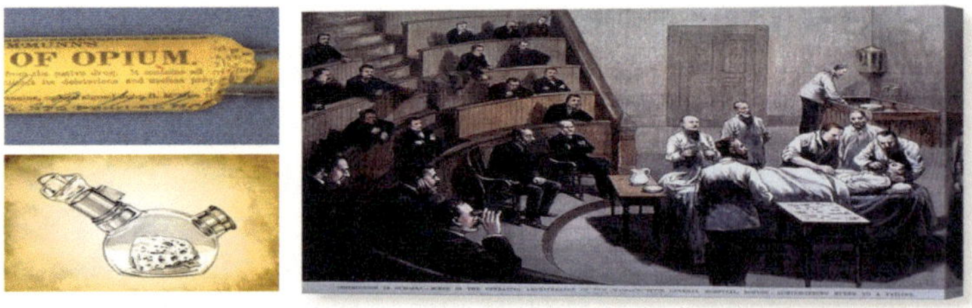


**Figure 1.**
*Preventing pain during surgery: From the use of opium poppy and other herbal remedies (early civilization) to the first public demonstration on October 16, 1846, at Massachusetts General Hospital (modern anesthesia). The history of anesthesia.*

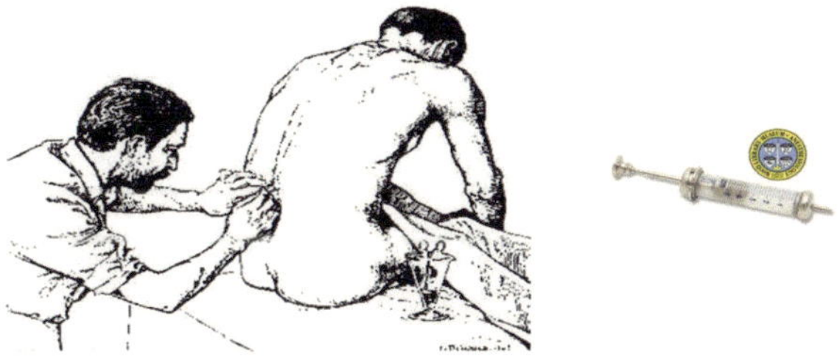

**Figure 2.**
*Epidural technique: Towards the improvement of needles and the refinement of local anesthetic.*

It was only from the end of the XIX century, with the development of needles and syringes, that allowed the introduction and safe use of regional anesthesia techniques epidural and spinal- with doctors F. Pagés and M. Dogliotti [8]. In the year 1899 and then at the year 1901 appeared the first publications on the use of spinal anesthesia and epidural anesthesia, respectively. Spinal techniques marked then a global milestone concept in the practice of anesthesia, at surgical activities but also in the developing of the Pain Units.

### 2.2 Overview about spinal anesthesia

Associated to the improving of the spinal technique (methods of performing, access route, dose, and the quality of the anesthetic substances) over time, the spinal pathway gained a prominent place, not only in the surgical field, but in other medical areas such as traumatology, rheumatology, pediatrics, internal medicine and oncology (**Figure 2**). Also, with the improvements of the spinal techniques, they reached the *gold standard* procedure in the Pain Units, as they allowed a continuous analgesia when necessary.

With the development of spinal techniques, injecting drugs into the epidural space is one of the most used interventions by anesthesiologists: local anesthetics, opioids, steroids, 'muscle relaxant'(baclofen), benzodiazepines (midazolam), clonidine, adenosine, ketamine, ziconotide, etc. Also, a specific mention to "hematic patch" in the management of post-dural puncture headache. In this way, the epidural space can be used, not only to provide anesthesia, but also to provide analgesia and to treating a variety of acute and chronic settings. In this context, the anesthesiologist should have a solid knowledge of the administered drugs within the epidural space.

Here we must add, then, another 'new drugs' to use into the epidural space: the biological therapies, the cell-based therapy.

## 3. Pathology of the medullary canal

Diseases engaged to the medullary canal, involved therefore to the epidural space, can be summarized as follows [9]:

1. Infection
2. Non-infectious medullary inflammation
3. Vertebromedullary trauma

4. Discovertebral degenerative processes

5. Inflammation of tumoral origin.

6. Postoperative spine

7. Congenital or acquired vascular pathology

It is not the aim of this chapter to deepen the study of the pathology of the medullary canal, but it is important to illustrate the changes that are linked to the degenerative processes of the discovertebral segment (number 4) in order to focus and understand what the vanguardist Regenerative Medicine therapy offers in the processes of the discovertebral impairment. In this regard, our goal is then to highlight the benefits of using the epidural space when we inject growth factors into the spinal segment. (Correa et al).

## 4. Degenerative disease of the spine

The spine is an articulated and highly resistant system, extending from the head to the pelvis. It plays a major role in protecting your body and supporting its movements. In between each vertebra of your spine lies an intervertebral disc. These discs allow the spine to generate movement and have flexibility. In addition, these discs serve as shock absorbers, protecting your vertebrae during everyday activities.

Spinal discs consist of a strong fibrous cartilage (the annulus fibrosus) which encloses a gel-like inner layer (the nucleus pulposus). As we age, these discs can weaken and become injured because of our personal habits, activities, diseases, and genetics. Degenerative disc disease is a painful degenerated disc. Degenerative disc disease is then an umbrella term that point out the pain that could extend from the neck to the lower back, associated with disc damage (**Figure 3**).

In the 1970s, Kirkaldy-Willis first described the "degenerative cascade" of the degenerative disc disease (DDD) (**Figure 4**) [10]. From an initial dysfunction of the disc, the fissure of the annulus fibrosus losing the capacity of containing the nucleus pulposus (first stage), to comprising the mobile segment, disc and facet joint degeneration leads to dynamic spinal instability (second stage), the patient finally develops a multifactorial stenosis, which may or may not be associated to instability (third stage) (**Figure 3**).

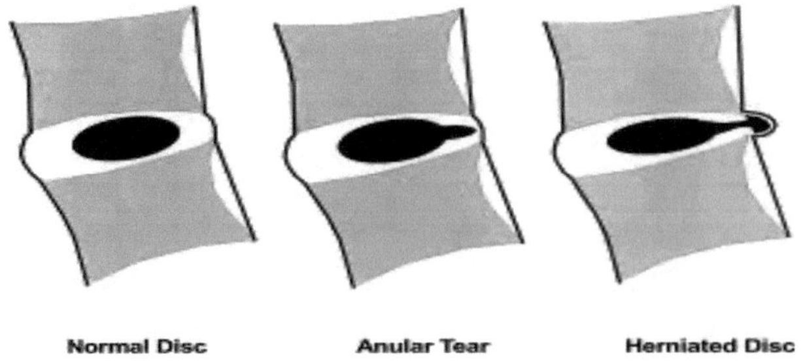


**Figure 3.**
*DDD: The evolution of the disc damage.*

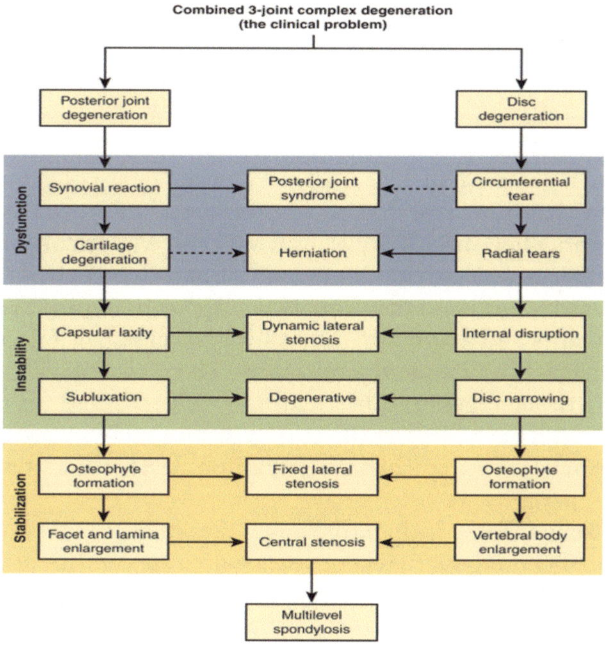


**Figure 4.**
*Kirkaldy-Willis spine: The "degenerative cascade".*

In this regard, the pathogenesis of the intervertebral disc disease process (IDD) involves a complex interplay of inflammatory, immunological, and pressure-related processes [11].

**In anatomical terms, intervertebral discs are the largest avascular structure of the body.**

Intervertebral disc, the flat, rubbery piece, that separate the bones of the backbones, have a very poor regenerative capacity [12]. Disc cells depend on the blood supply at the margins of the discs for their nutrients. The nucleus and inner anulus of the disc are supplied by capillaries that arise in the vertebral bodies, penetrate the subchondral bone, and terminate at the bone-disc junction. Despite being highly implicated in disc degeneration, the end plate has hardly been quoted into regenerative strategies [13, 14].

Current therapeutic approaches should therefore be focused on combating the disc's poor nutritional supply, diffused from the blood vessels of the vertebral body through the cartilaginous end plate. However, the current treatments for IDD, proposed in most ´consensus protocols´ do not correspond to the pathophysiological process involved in the IDD, as these treatments are mainly focused on relieving pain (palliative pain medicine). Surgical techniques (including fusion, laminectomy, and discectomy), aim to stabilize the spine and/or decompress the spinal or the foraminal canal thus alleviating symptoms, but these techniques are not addressed to regarding the cause of the degeneration, and sometimes even accelerate the degeneration of the adjacent segments.

**So, it is only through the understanding of the spine pathophysiology and its clinical course that will allow us to provide a rational treatment for patients.**

At present, treatment options for degenerative disc disease remain suboptimal, and development and outcomes of novel treatment options currently must be considered unpredictable.

## 5. Understanding platelet-rich plasma (PRP)

The biology of platelet-rich plasma and its effect in the process of healing is a promising biological therapeutic strategy for enhance the regenerative process and healing of the damaged tissue (**Figure 5**).

The regenerative potential of PRP is based on the release of growth factors that occurs with platelet rupture. The first clinical report of PRP used as tissue regenerative therapy was published in 1998 by an oral surgeon who incorporates PRP into spongy bone grafting to reconstruct large mandibular defects [15]. Since then, PRP has been widely used in oral and maxillofacial surgery to improve osseointegration of dental implants and accelerate the healing process [16, 17]. More recently it has been used to treat injuries to the musculoskeletal system. Thus, at present, the use of PRP as a tissue regeneration therapy is well accepted for its modulating and stimulating properties of cell proliferation of mesenchymal origin (fibroblasts, osteoblasts, endothelial cells, epithelial cells, adipoblasts, myocytes and chondrocytes, mainly).

Platelet Rich Plasma (PRP) is then, the novel therapeutic tool of autologous nature that is strongly emerging in recent years with a successful therapeutic use. Different PRP studies have showed a beneficial effect on the target cells, which allows to propose its use the treatment of several pathological processes: the healing of wounds, the processes of tissue regeneration, or in the treatment of cellular involution that takes place with aging [18]. Clinically, PRP has been shown to decrease pain and increase function in chronic elbow tendinosis patients. PRP has also been used in plantar fasciitis, spinal fusion, and in total knee arthroplasty with varying degrees of success. PRP accelerated wound healing of human skin punch wounds in a recent prospective, controlled study.

**In conclusion, the rationale behind the use of PRP is the deliver a high concentrations of growth factors and cytokines which can improve the healing process.**

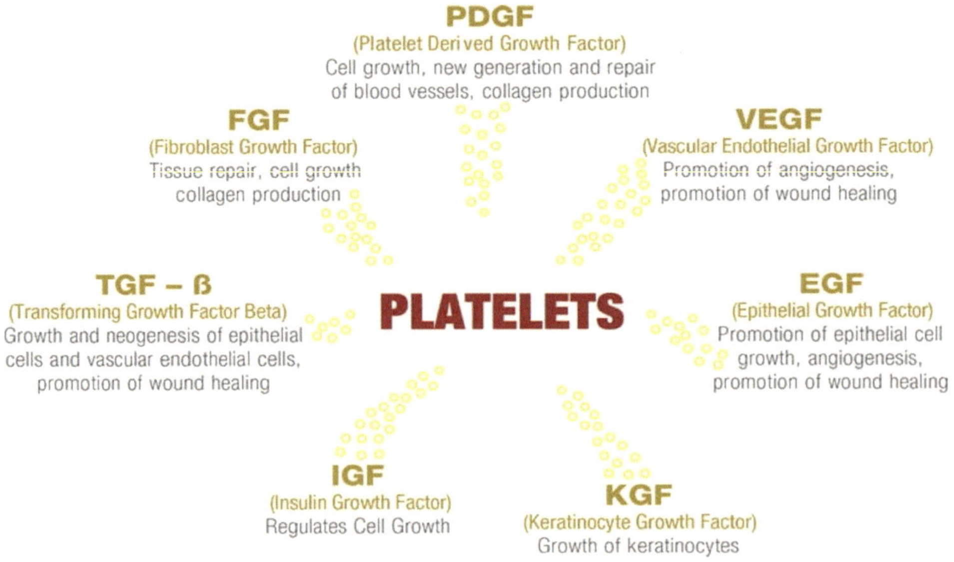


**Figure 5.**
*Platelet-rich plasma: Growth factors and pro- and anti-inflammatory properties.*

### 5.1 Tissue and cicatrization engineering around PRP

#### *5.1.1 Regeneration: the healing process*

Plasma rich in growth factors (PRGF) is a recent cell-based technique being evaluated for promoting tissue healing, as PRGF has shown in vitro and in vivo the potential to stimulate matrix metabolism [19–24]. Upon activation, these platelets release a variety of cell signaling molecules such as platelet-derived growth factor (PDGF), insulin-like growth factor (IGF-1), transforming grow factor (TGF-β1), vascular endothelial growth factor (VEGF), hepatocyte growth factor (HGF) and basic fibroblastic growth factor (FGF). Other mediators, nerve growth factor (NGF), brain-derived neurotrophic factor (BDNF), and other neurotropic factors such as fibrin, fibronectin, and vitronectin, are also activated [24–26]. All these plasma biological mediators govern tissue repair although their mechanisms of action in the healing process are still poorly understood.

#### *5.1.2 The anti-inflammatory effect with PRGF*

Evidence suggests that biomolecules conveyed by PRGFs are instrumental agents that modulate early inflammation [27], also involved in the macrophage polarization, angiogenesis, and fibrogenesis, the stem cell-like myelinating SC activation, and finally, they have an active rol in the resolution of inflammation. Considering this benefit (anti-inflammatory effect) on the spinal axis intrathecal administration of transforming growth factor β1 (TGF-β1), a potent anti-inflammatory cytokine, has demonstrated to alleviate nerve injury- induced neuropathic pain in rats, attenuating nerve injury-induced neuropathic pain [28]. TGF-β1 acted as a powerful neuromodulator and rapidly (within minutes) suppressed chronic constriction injury–evoked spinal synaptic plasticity and dorsal root ganglion neuronal hyperexcitability, alleviating early- and late- phase neuropathic pain symptoms, such as allodynia and hyperalgesia, for several weeks in murine models. These previous studies -in murine models-, allowed us to raise the hypothesis that PRP could help us to relieve neuropathic pain that is associated with DDD [29].

#### *5.1.3 The neuroprotective effect of PRGF*

Several growth factors present in plasma including the nerve growth factor (NGF), brain derivate neurotrophic factor (BDNF), PDGF, VEGF, IGF-1, transforming growth factor beta (TGFB) alone or in combination have been shown to exert an antiapoptotic and neuroprotective effect on mesenchymal stem cells (MSCs), neurons, the Schwann cells (SCs), and human neural stem cells [25, 30].

## 6. Epidural PRP

The clinical evidence for PRGF treatment of discogenic low back pain in humans was reported in 2011 [31]. Since then, many research papers, in vitro and in vivo studies, have confirmed the efficacy of PRGF in IDD management. However, early in vivo studies used intradiscal injection of PRGF. These early documents concluded that intradiscal injection of autologous PRGF in patients with low back pain is safe and free of adverse events [29–33]. However, the intradiscal injection of PRGF technique is a more laborious proceeding and probably limits the effects. The first document injecting PRP into the epidural space was our paper [4]. Knowing the biology of platelet-rich plasma and its restorative effect on cartilages (in general) and its repairing effect on the vertebral disc (in particular) allowed us to propose the use of PRP into the epidural space.

### 6.1 Why PDGF into the epidural space?

The choice of the epidural space needs a good knowledge of its anatomy and its content, as well as the pharmacodynamics of the medication we are using.

The first published study using the epidural space while injecting PRGF was our paper [4]. Our first line of work was only a clinical trial, assessing the pain relief response and assessing the degree of functional recovery of the patient. Our reason for changing the intradiscal injection technique, preferring the epidural space was that, compared to intradiscal injection, growth factors by epidural route would fulfill an effective outcome by acting not only on the discs, but also over the facet joints and the ligamentum flavum, and, because of its anti-inflammatory activity. That further study had allowed us to confirm that this technique -epidural PRP- help with relieving the neuropathic pain (NP) associated to IDD [29].

### 6.2 Axial structure: the "poly-articular component"

We have considered the axial region as a "multi-articular component", where the epidural space would be an ideal place to inject PRP (**Figure 6**). The epidural space will allow us to reach the intervertebral disc, but also the facet joint, and even more, we can get the benefit of PRP in the foraminal region. Thus, the epidural space permits a pharmacological manipulation of various segments of this region, considering its inter-cellular signaling pathway.

### 6.3 Plasma rich in growth factors: the chemical signaling

Inter-cellular signaling is the communication between cells. The main difference between the different categories of signaling is the distance that the signal travels

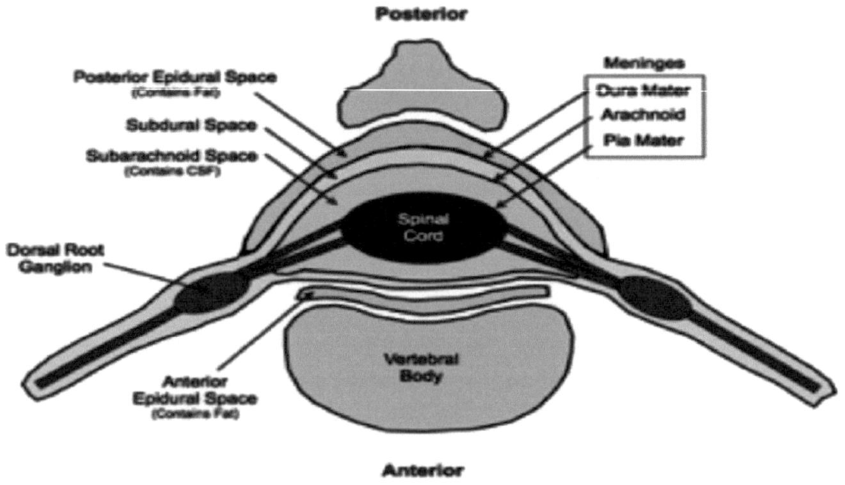


**Figure 6.**
*Anatomy of the axial region.*

through the organism to reach the target cell. In chemical signaling, a cell may target itself (autocrine signaling), a cell connected by gap junctions, a nearby cell (paracrine signaling), or a distant cell (endocrine signaling).

Multiple studies have demonstrated a beneficial effect of many of these growth factors, e.g., platelet-derived growth factors (PDGFs), fibroblast growth factors (FGFs), and granulocyte-macrophage colony stimulating factor (GM-CSF) on the healing process, accelerating wound closure with increased reepithelialization, cell infiltration, granulation formation, and angiogenesis. In all stages of the repair, a wide variety of different growth factors and cytokines are involved. The release of these various growth factors, cytokines, and low-molecular-weight compounds from degranulating platelets, are the mediators for the healing process. Fibroblasts, osteoblasts, endothelial cells, leukocytes, monocytes, and macrophages are cells involved in the produce of growth factors.

**Growth factors and cytokines work as paracrine signals, that means they act locally, between cells that are close together** [34].

With these two concepts in mind (the axial structure and the way to act of the PRP) we considered that growth factors by epidural route would fulfill our expecting outcome.

Using PRGF in patients with IDD was considered, few years ago, merely as another "off the shelf" alternative. Recent studies, and our clinical results, now we have a different opinion: PRGFs should be the "flagship" within in the multimodal therapeutic scheme for IDD. Accumulated evidence, in both preclinical and clinical settings, indicates that PRGF and fibrin scaffold have an important therapeutic role in patients with IDD: (1) its potential to enhancing cartilage regeneration, (2) reducing the catabolic factors that lead to cartilage degradation, (3) its neuroinflammatory therapeutic modulation, (4) its neuroprotective effect. With these effects in mind, we achieve the sensory and motor functional recovery. However, only a few cell-based clinical trials targeting IDD repair or regeneration have been published, and most of them use axial PRP through intradiscal injection. Also, none of them have the long-term necessary MRI study in the clinical follow-up. In our understanding, we decide to use the biological therapy by the epidural approaching in the management of IDD. Injecting PRP into the epidural space means cytokines (inflammation control) and high concentrations of growth factors (tissue repair and regeneration). Epidural PRP allows us to suggest this is the first-line technique in the healing process of IDD.

**PRP is a rich source of growth factors that promote tissue regeneration. Also, PRP suppress cytokine release, limiting inflammation, improving thereby, the healing process. So, Epidural PRP allows us to suggest this is the first-line technique in managing IDD.**

### 6.4 Our designed study with PRP within the epidural space

The preliminary study, a clinical trial in which PRGF was injected into the epidural space for promoting IDD regeneration, started since 2014, and published in 2016 [4]. That preliminary trial included 70 patients, and they were injected with one epidural PRGF dose. That pilot trial focused on clinical perspectives (pain relief and assessment of patient satisfaction through VAS score and Macnab criteria).

Then, a new and larger study [5] reached 250 patients who received two doses of epidural PRP and who were assessed with magnetic resonance imaging (MRI) one year after PRP treatment to find disc or facet join changes if they occurred. That was probably the most extensive follow-up document that links PRGF used in injection into the epidural space as a method of intervertebral disc regeneration in cases of disc disease, and the only one with MRI evaluation before PRGF treatment, and then one year posterior to the PRGF therapy.

Even considering that it was a field of research, still in early development, our novel alternative treatment with promising clinical results for intervertebral disc disorders was far distant from the poor results usually achieved with previous consensus protocols, those based on palliative pain medications, but not focused on treating the underlying disease.

### 6.5 Design of the second study

Prospective observational, nonrandomized, single-center clinical study carried out between January 2015 and June 2017. We have included 250 patients, who were between 18 years to 70 years of age, with neck or back pain with or without radicular pain, and with a diagnosis of a spinal disc herniation confirmed with MRI imaging. After receiving institutional approval and informed consent signed by all patients, they were approached for enrollment. In the majority of patients, the etiopathogenesis of the axial or radicular pain was due to multifactorial origin: disc disease, facet joint arthrosis, hypertrophy of the ligamentum flavum, and in many cases associated to central canal narrowing or foraminal stenosis.

### 6.6 Results of the preliminary study

Epidural PRGF injections for IDD showed clinically significant improvements in pain (VAS-scale) and function (MACNAB-score) (**Table 1**) throughout two years of follow-up.

Mean VAS-scale improved in 85% of patients, from 9 to 3, and the mean MACNAB-score was considered GOOD at six months and EXCELLENT at the end of one year after the epidural PRGF injections. The need for opioid rescue decreased from 96% to none at the end of one year follow-up (**Table 2**). However, 15% of the patients did not improve the pain score; but no patient showed a worsening of the symptoms. Positive changes in MRI images one year following the second epidural dose have been documented in few patients, but this aspect needs further research.

With these results, our pilot study showed a definitive role of PRP injection via the epidural space for chronic prolapsed intervertebral disc patients.

| |
|---|
| **1. Excellent:** No pain. No restriction of mobility. Return to normal work and level of activity. |
| **2. Good:** Relief of current symptoms. Occasional back or leg pain of sufficient severity to interfere with the patient's ability to do his normal work or his capacity to enjoy himself in his leisure hours. Able to return to modified work. |
| **3. Fair:** Improved functional capacity but handicapped by intermittent pain of sufficient severity to curtail or modify work or leisure activities. Still handicapped and/or unemployed. |
| **4. Poor:** No improvement or insufficient improvement to enable increasing activities. Continued objective symptoms of root involvement. Probable further operative intervention needed, irrespective of length of postoperative follow-up. |

**Table 1.**
*Modified Macnab criteria.*

| Outcome assessment | VAS scale | MACNAB score | Opioid rescue |
|---|---|---|---|
| Previous to PRGF injection | 9/10 | POOR | 96% of patients |
| Two months after two doses of PRGF | 4/10 | FAIR | 20% of patients |
| Six months after two doses of PRGF | 3/10 | GOOD | none |
| One year after two doses of PRGF | 2/10 | EXCELLENT | none |

**Table 2.**
*Outcome of patients after epidural PRGF injections.*

## 7. Conclusions

1. Consensuses, in general, need to be updated periodically [35].

2. Pain Units are having great changes. Palliative management of pain has specific indications, but far from the goal of managing osteoarticular degenerative diseases. Mere palliative management of pain in osteoarticular degenerative disease is then, the second line option. Introducing the development of Regenerative Medicine (RM), regenerative therapies (mesenchymal stem cells and many growth factors from stem cells) which allow to promote and improve the healing process, may become a new current therapeutic method for healing in the future, and of course, a wide reception and a wide cover in pain units.

3. Low back pain (LBP) is a major public health issue. A thorough understanding of the pathophysiology and clinical manifestations is necessary to focusing a solid treatment.

4. In the management of the intervertebral disc disease (IDD), there are three headings: (1) Relief of pain by conservative management (physiotherapy, oral analgesia and supplements, alternative medicine); (2) Restorative treatment of the intervertebral disc (growth factor therapy, molecular or cell therapy) according to the principles of tissue engineering, (3) Surgery (decompression or total disc replacement, or rigid fusion surgery when necessary). With this in mind, the approach to IDD requires a multimodal technique in its management. Unfortunately, most conservative therapies and spinal surgeries are only aimed to relieve the symptoms, but do not address the cause of the degeneration. Even more, surgery techniques could accelerate the degeneration of adjacent segments.

5. Tissue regeneration strategies such as tissue engineering, growth factor administration, and stem cell-based therapies, have undergone significant development over the past two decades. Regenerative medicine, from tissue engineering to cell therapy, offers valuable treatment options, but sadly, they are rarely considered in daily clinical settings.

6. Growth factors have been enjoying more popularity in the field of regeneration of IDD and many have been proved to be effective in reversing the degenerative trend of the intervertebral disc. In this point, the epidural space is, in our opinion, the best option to perform this technique, as using this route -the

epidural space- will allow an effective activity on the disc, but also over the facet joints, and on the ligamentum flavum. Its antineuroinflammatory activity would relieve the associated neuropathic pain.

7. Finally, in IDD, the regenerative medicine option, such as the use of mesenchymal stem cells or platelet-rich plasma, has shown preclinical and clinical positive results. However, additional more powered high-quality studies are needed to really appreciate the long-term safety and efficacy of this technique approaches in the IDD process.

## Author details

José Correa[1*], Henry Cortés[2], Lucia Correa[3] and Rita López[1]

1 Hospital Santiago Apóstol, Miranda de Ebro, Spain

2 Pain Management-Palliative Care, Medical Cannabis Global Health Initiative Specialist, Spain

3 IQS, Universitat Ramon Llull, Barcelona, Spain

*Address all correspondence to: josep24909@hotmail.com

## References

[1] Shvartzman L, Weingarten E, Sherry H, Levin S, Persaud A. Cost-effectiveness analysis of extended conservative therapy versus surgical intervention in the management of herniated lumbar intervertebral disc. Spine. 1992;**15**:176-182

[2] Frymoyer JW, Cats-Baril WL. An overview of the incidence and costs of low back pain. The Orthopedic Clinics of North America. 1991;**15**:263-271

[3] Wu PH, Kim HS, Jang IT. Intervertebral disc diseases PART 2: A review of the current diagnostic and treatment strategies for intervertebral disc disease. International Journal of Molecular Sciences. 2020;**21**(6):2135. DOI: 10.3390/ijms21062135

[4] Correa J, Cortés H, Coral O, García E. PRP epidural en el manejo de la enfermedad discal degenerativa y dolor axial. Estudio preliminar. Rev. Soc. Esp. Dolor. 2017;**24**(2):85-95

[5] Jose C, Henry C, Patricia A, Edwin G. Epidural plasma rich in growth factors for degenerative disc disease: A valuable alternative to conventional "palliative medicine". International Journal of Anesthesia and Clinical Medicine. 2019;**7**(1):1-6. DOI: 10.11648/j.ijacm.20190701.11

[6] Bhatia R, Chopra G. Efficacy of platelet rich plasma via lumbar epidural route in chronic prolapsed intervertebral disc patients-a pilot study. Journal of Clinical and Diagnostic Research. 2016;**10**(9):UC05-UC07. DOI: 10.7860/JCDR/2016/21863.8482

[7] WLM Library – Free eBooks: https://www.woodlibrarymuseum.org/e-book/the-history-of-anesthesiology-reprint-series

[8] Gonzalo Rodríguez V, Rivero Martínez D, Pérez Albacete M, López López A, Maluff TA. Historia de la Raquianestesia y de la Anestesia Epidural en España. Archivos Españoles de Urología. 2007;**60**(8):973-978

[9] Boleaga DB. Patología inflamatoria de la columna vertebral. Anales de Radiología México. 2005;**2**:105-114

[10] Kirkaldy-Willis WH, Wedge JH, Yong-Hing K, Reilly J. Pathology and pathogenesis of lumbar spondylosis and stenosis. Spine. 1978;**3**:319

[11] Molinos M, Almeida CR, Caldeira J, Cunha C, Gonçalves RM, Barbosa MA. Inflammation in intervertebral disc degeneration and regeneration. J R Soc Interface. 2015;**(6)**; **12 (104)**:20141191

[12] Smith LJ, Nerurkar NL, Choi K-S, Harfe BD, Elliott DM. Degeneration and regeneration of the intervertebral disc: Lessons from development. Disease Models & Mechanisms. 2011 Jan;**4**(1):31-41

[13] Moore RJ. The vertebral endplate: disc degeneration, disc regeneration. European Spine Journal. 2006;**15**(Suppl. 3): 333-337

[14] Wang Y, Videman T, Battie MC. ISSLS prize winner: Lumbar vertebral endplate lesions: Associations with disc degeneration and back pain history. Spine. 2012;**37**(17):1490-1496

[15] Marx RE, Carlson ER, Eichstaedt RM, Schimmele SR, Strauss JE, Georgeff KR. Platelet-rich plasma: Growth fac- tor enhancement for bone grafts. Oral Surgery, Oral Medicine, Oral Pathology, Oral Radiology, and Endodontics. 1998;**85**(6):638-646

[16] Arora NS, Ramanayake T, Ren YF, Romanos GE. Platelet- rich plasma in sinus augmentation procedures: A systematic literature review: Part II. Implant Dentistry. 2010;**19**(2):145-157. DOI: 10.1097/ID.0b013e3181cd706d

[17] Del Fabbro M, Bortolin M, Taschieri S, Weinstein R. Is platelet concentrate advantageous for the surgical treatment of periodontal diseases? A systematic review and meta-analysis. Journal of Periodontology. 2011;**82**(8):1100-1111. DOI: 10.1902/jop.2010.100605

[18] Wang SZ, Rui YF, Tan Q, Wang C. Enhancing intervertebral disc repair and regeneration through biology: Platelet-rich plasma as an alternative strategy. Arthritis Research & Therapy. 2013;**15**(5):220. DOI: 10.1186/ar4353

[19] Nguyen RT, Borg-Stein J, Mcinnis K. Application of platelet- rich plasma in musculoskeletal and sports medicine: An evidence-based approach. PM & R: The Journal of Injury, Function, and Rehabilitation. 2011;**3**:226-250

[20] Molloy T, Wang Y, Murrell G. The roles of growth factors in tendon and ligament healing. Sports Medicine. 2003;**33**:381-394

[21] Rodríguez J, Palomar MA, Torres J. Plasma rico en plaquetas: fundamentos biológicos y aplicaciones en cirugía maxilofacial y estética facial. Rev Esp Cirug Oral y Maxilofac. 2012;**34**(1):8-17

[22] Marx RE, Carlson ER, Eichstaedt RM, Schimmele SR, Strauss JE, Georgeff KR. Platelet-rich plasma: Growth factor enhancement for bone grafts. Oral Surgery, Oral Medicine, Oral Pathology, Oral Radiology, and Endodontics. 1998;**85**(6):638-646

[23] Lubkowska A, Dolegowska B, Banfi G. Growth factor content in PRP and their applicability in medicine. Journal of Biological Regulators and Homeostatic Agents. 2012;**26**(2 Suppl. 1): 3S-22S

[24] Sánchez M, Anitua E, Delgado D, Sanchez P, Prado R, Orive G, et al. Platelet-rich plasma, a source of autologous growth factors and biomimetic scaffold for peripheral nerve regeneration. Expert Opinion on Biological Therapy. 2017;**17**(2):197-212

[25] Sánchez M, Garate A, Delgado D, Padilla S. Platelet-rich plasma, an adjuvant biological therapy to assist peripheral nerve repair. Neural Regeneration Research. 2017;**12**(1): 47-52

[26] Anitua E, Pelacho B, Prado R, Aguirre JJ, Sánchez M, Padilla S, et al. Infiltration of plasma rich in growth factors enhances in vivo angiogenesis and improves reperfusion and tissueremodeling after severe hind limb ischemia. Journal of Controlled Release. 2015d;**202**:31-39

[27] El-Sharkawy H, Kantarci A, Deady J, Hasturk H, Liu H, Alshahat M, et al. Platelet-rich plasma: Growth factors and pro- and anti-inflammatory properties. Journal of Periodontology. 2007;**78**(4):661-669

[28] Echeverry S, Shi XQ, Haw A, Liu H, Zhang Z, Zhang J. Transforming growth factor-β1 impairs neuropathic pain through pleiotropic effects. Molecular Pain. 2009;**5**:16. DOI: 10.1186/17448069-5-16

[29] Correa J, Cortés H, García E, Quintero L. Platelet-rich plasma in treating peripheral neuropathic pain. Preliminary report (Plasma rico en plaquetas en el tratamiento del dolor neuropático periférico. Estudio preliminary). Rev. Soc. Esp. Dolor.

2018;**25**(5):263-270. DOI: 10.20986/resed.2017.3625/2017

[30] Blobe GC, Schiemann WP, Lodish HF. Role of transforming growth factor beta in human disease. The New England Journal of Medicine. 2000;**342**:1350-1358. DOI: 10.1056/NEJM200005043421807

[31] Akeda K, Imanishi T, Ohishi K, et al. Intradiscal Injection of Autologous Serum Isolated from Platelet-Rich-Plasma for the Treatment of Discogenic Low Back Pain: Preliminary Prospective Clinical Trial: GP141. Spine: Affiliated Society Meeting Abstracts; 2011

[32] Monfett M, Harrison J, Boachie-Adjei K, Lutz G. Intradiscal platelet-rich plasma (PRP) injections for discogenic low back pain: An update. International Orthopaedics. 2016;**40**(6):1321-1328

[33] Tuakli-Wosornu YA, Terry A, Boachie-Adjei K, et al. Lumbar Intradiskal platelet-rich plasma (PRP) injections: A prospective, double-blind. Randomized Controlled Study. PM R. 2016;**8**:1-10

[34] Yew TL, Hung YT, Li HY, Chen HW, Chen LL, Tsai KS, et al. Enhancement of wound healing by human multipotent stromal cell conditioned medium: The paracrine factors and p38 MAPK activation. CellTransplant. 2011;**20**(5):693-706. DOI: 10.3727/096368910X550198

[35] J. Correa, P Abella. Unidades del dolor del siglo XXI. ¿Protocolos de consenso o medicina basada en la evidencia? (21st Century Pain Units: Consensus Protocols or Evidence-Based Medicine?) Revista Persona y bioética de la Universidad de la Sabana, Bogotá. ISSN-e 0123-3122, 22, 1, 2018. 29-38

Section 4

# Epidural Administration and the ICU

Chapter 6

# Epidural Analgesia for Pain Management in the Intensive Care Unit

*Kingsley U. Tobi*

## Abstract

The pain of patients admitted into the ICU remains poorly reported and managed. It has been reported that about half of patients admitted to both medical and surgical ICU experienced significant pain during their stay in the unit. Most of these patients tend to develop psycho-traumatic experiences both while in the unit and after discharge. This chapter thus highlights the drawback of poor pain management of critically ill patients and the role of epidural analgesia in contributing to better pain control in the ICU.

**Keywords:** epidural analgesia, pain, critically ill, ICU, pain management

## 1. Introduction

Pain, as defined by the International Association for the study of pain, is an unpleasant sensory and emotional experience associated with actual or potential tissue damage or described in terms of such damage [1]. It is common among patients in the intensive care unit (ICU). Previously, a prospective study reported that about half of patients admitted to both medical and surgical ICU experienced significant pain during their stay in the unit [2]. Although most ICU patients cannot self-report pain, its presence often leads to deleterious consequences during and after discharge from the unit. Adequate pain control in the ICU is essential and adds to optimal patient care with improved outcomes.

The pain of patients admitted into the ICU remains poorly reported and managed. Most of these patients as a result tend to develop psycho-traumatic experiences both while in the unit and after discharge. This chapter thus highlights the drawback of poor pain management of critically ill patients and the role of epidural analgesia in contributing to better pain control in the ICU.

## 2. Aetiology of pain in ICU

The aetiology of pain among ICU patients ranges from injuries sustained prior to admission, postoperative pain, pain due to patient's pathology and pain during routine nursing procedures such as turning, wound dressing and suctioning. A significant increase in pain intensity during patient turning in the ICU compared to when they were lying down at rest has also been documented [3].

## 3. Impact of pain on ICU patients

Poor or inadequate pain relief in the intensive care unit has a multi-systemic impact on the critically ill patient. Suboptimal pain management in the ICU can lead to anxiety, delirium and sleep deprivation. Anxiety leads to agitation, patient-ventilator asynchrony and difficulty in weaning from the ventilator [4]. Inadequate pain relief can lead to improper sleep, and lack of adequate sleep can increase pain response in ICU patients.

Furthermore, inadequate analgesia in the ICU is associated with increased oxygen consumption and sympathetic responses with increased poor outcomes. In mechanically ventilated patients, pain may lead to retained pulmonary secretions, resulting in secondary bacteria colonisation and the development of ventilator-associated pneumonia (VAP) [5]. Ventilator-associated pneumonia complicates ICU management, with an increased risk of morbidity and mortality.

In addition, poor pain control in the ICU can often lead to post-traumatic stress disorder (PTSD). Granja and colleagues found that about two out of ten ICU patients experience severe pain six months after being discharged from the unit [4]. This can lead to chronic pain with its attendant psychosocial and economic burden on the patients, family members and the health care system.

The stress response following, for example, surgical intervention causes an increase in stress hormones in the circulation. This can result in arteriolar vasoconstriction, impair tissue perfusion, and reduce tissue-oxygen partial pressure [6]. The consequences include poor wound healing and surgical wound infection [7], resulting in poor patient outcomes in the ICU.

## 4. Pain assessment in the ICU

Most patients admitted to the ICU cannot correctly communicate the intensity of their pain. This may be due to a reduced level of consciousness and the different interventions provided, such as airway and ventilatory support [8]. Since the inability to report pain does not exclude its presence [9], the need to properly assess pain intensity among ICU patients cannot be overemphasised.

Due to patients' inability to communicate their pain, behavioural and physical responses have been used to assess pain in the ICU. The two commonly employed behavioural pain assessment tools used in sedated and ventilated patients are the Behavioural Pain Scale (BPS) and Critical-Care Pain Observation Tool (CPOT) [10]. The BPS is a clinical observational score depending upon the patient's facial expressions, upper limb posturing, and tolerance of the controlled mechanical ventilation. The score ranges from 3 to 12, and a score of >6 requires pain management [10].

See **Table 1** below:

| | | |
|---|---|---|
| | Relaxed | 1 |
| Facial expressions | Partially tightened | 2 |
| | Fully tight | 3 |
| | Grimacing | 4 |
| | No movements | 1 |
| | Partially bent | 2 |
| Upper limbs | Fully bent with fingers flexion | 3 |
| | Permanently retracted | 4 |
| | Tolerating movements | 1 |
| Compliance with mechanical ventilation | Coughing but tolerating ventilation most of the time | 2 |
| | Fighting with ventilator | 3 |
| | Unable to control the ventilation | 4 |

**Table 1.**
*Behavioural pain scale (BPS).*

The Critical-care Pain Observation Tool is a pain assessment tool with four clinical components, facial expressions, body movements and muscle tension and compliance with invasive mechanical ventilation. The score ranges from 2 to 8, and a score of more than 2 requires pain management intervention. See **Table 2**:

| **Sub-scale** | **Description** | **Score** |
|---|---|---|
| | Relaxed, neutral | 0 |
| Facial expression | Tense | 1 |
| | Grimacing | 2 |
| | Absence of movements | 0 |
| Body movements | Protection | 1 |
| | Restlessness | 1 |
| | Relaxed | 0 |
| Muscle tension | Tense, rigid | 1 |
| | Very tense or rigid | 2 |
| | Tolerating ventilator or movement | 0 |
| Compliance with ventilation | Coughing but tolerating | 1 |
| | Fighting ventilator | 2 |
| | Talking in normal tone or no sound | 0 |
| Vocalisation (extubated patients) | Sighing, moaning | 1 |
| | Crying out, sobbing | 2 |

**Table 2.**
*Critical-care pain observation tool (CPOT).*

In our setting, the Behavioural Pain Scale (BPS) is easier to use and, when combined with other clinical observations, helps to determine the adequacy of analgesia in our patients.

## 5. Pain management in the ICU

One of the methods of achieving pain control in the ICU is via epidural analgesia. Epidural analgesia/anaesthesia is a form of neuraxial block where local anaesthetic agents and other adjuvants, such as opioids, are deposited into the epidural space. This may be done as a single-shot technique or with a catheter or continuous infusion. It offers a wide range of applications and may be performed at the cervical, thoracic, lumbar and sacral levels.

In a survey conducted in England, 89% of ICUs use epidurals for pain relief [11]. There are, however, some concerns about "the safety of placing epidural catheters in sedated patients, and confirmation of a good catheter position can be difficult in the critically ill patient if sensory level testing is not reliable" [12]. Apart from the safety concerns raised with epidural analgesia in the ICU, placing an epidural catheter in critically ill patients is sometimes difficult. This may be due to difficulty with properly positioning patients for the procedure, presence of contraindications such as sepsis and coagulopathy, common in ICU patients and the haemodynamic complications following the procedure. With the availability of trained personnel and improved monitoring, epidural analgesia can be safely done for appropriate patients in the ICU.

## 6. Anatomy of the epidural space

The epidural space is a potential space between the dural sheath and the spinal canal. It is continuous within the vertebral column and extends from the foramen magnum to the sacrococcygeal membrane of the sacral canal [13]. The foramen magnum occupies the superior boundary, and the sacral hiatus occupies the inferior boundary. The posterior longitudinal ligament and ligamentum flavum form the anterior and posterior boundaries, respectively. The vertebral laminae, pedicles and intervertebral foramen form the lateral boundary.

Some of the contents of the epidural space include semi-liquid fats (extra-dural fats), lymphatics, arteries and large thin-walled veins. The capacity of the epidural space is far greater than the capacity of the subarachnoid space. It requires 1.5–2.0 mls of LA to block a spinal segment via the epidural route against 0.3 mls via the subarachnoid space.

The veins within the epidural space constitute a close network which runs vertically. They form four (4) main trunks, namely: two (2) on either side of the posterior longitudinal ligament and two (2) posteriorly in front of the vertebral arches. The epidural veins anastomose freely with extra-dural veins, the azygous veins and the intracranial veins. The veins are called valveless venous plexus of Bateson.

The epidural space has a negative pressure transmitted intra-pleural pressure via the thoracic paravertebral space. This negative pressure may also be due to the relative overgrowth of the vertebral canal compared with the dural sac. Artefactual or transient negative pressure results from the needle's anterior dimpling of the dural. It can also arise from the anterior indentation of the ligamentum flavum by the epidural needle. In addition, back flexion causes stretching of the dural sac and pushes CSF out.

## 7. Indications for epidural Analgesia in the ICU

Indications for epidural Analgesia in the ICU include [12]:

- Blunt trauma with or without rib fractures
- Surgical such as thoracic, abdominal, orthopaedic, cardiac and vascular surgeries
- Non-surgical indications such as intractable angina pectoris and acute pancreatitis

## 8. Contraindications for epidural Analgesia

These could be absolute or relative. Absolute contraindications include:

- Patient refusal
- Infection at the proposed catheter insertion site
- Sepsis
- Hypovolemia (shock)
- Allergy to local anaesthetic agents and opioids.

Relative contraindications include:

- Coagulopathy
- Increased intracranial pressure
- Neurological disorder
- Spine deformity

## 9. Technique for epidural Analgesia

Three methods can be used to administer epidural analgesia in the ICU: single-injection and intermittent boluses, continuous infusion via an indwelling catheter or patient-controlled epidural analgesia (PCEA). Continuous infusion via an indwelling catheter is often preferred in the ICU because it offers a constant plasma level of administered analgesics, thus providing better and more efficacious pain relief [13].

The following are steps to performing an epidural in the ICU.

*Patient selections:* Most surgical patients admitted to the intensive care units postoperatively in which epidural anaesthesia was provided would have an epidural catheter in situ. Others who do not already have one are selected based on a careful assessment of patient status, risks, benefits, indications and contraindications of epidural analgesia.

*Patient consent:* After careful patient selection, informed consent should be obtained from the patient if awake or from the relative before proceeding with the technique. Informed consent should involve a careful explanation of the procedure and the risks and benefits of the procedure. Consent may be in the form of written or verbal.

*Positioning:* epidural analgesia can be done with the patient sitting or lateral decubitus. However, in the ICU, the commoner position for an epidural is the lateral decubitus position due to the peculiarities of ICU patients. With the patient in the appropriate position, an epidural needle, typically a Tuohy needle, is inserted into the appropriate intervertebral space to the epidural space aseptically. Correct placement is confirmed with a loss of resistance or hanging drop technique.

*Placement of catheter:* Following confirmation of the correct needle placement in the epidural space, an epidural catheter may be threaded into the epidural space through the Touhy or spinal needle for a continuous top-up. The epidural catheter is advanced 2–3 cm into the epidural space [14], after which the needle is carefully removed. A slide-lock adapter may be attached to the end of the catheter to allow the attachment of an injection port or infusion tubing. A filter can also be attached to the infusion tubing to ensure sterility. The placement of an epidural catheter is determined by the dermatome innervating the area of pain to be treated. On the other, an epidural catheter can be placed directly at the site of injury or at the site of surgical incision.

*Prevention of intrathecal or vascular injection:* Two techniques are used to prevent the intrathecal and/or vascular placement of an epidural catheter, namely, aspiration and the use of a test dose. For the aspiration method, a syringe filled with two millilitres of preservative-free sterile normal saline is attached to the end of the catheter and gently aspirated for 30 seconds. A bloody tap implies that the catheter is in an epidural vein. In addition, an increase in heart rate or blood pressure following a test dose of a local anaesthetic with 1:200,000 adrenaline indicates that the tip of the catheter may be in an epidural vein. More than one millilitre of clear fluid which is positive for cerebrospinal fluid shows that the catheter is in the subarachnoid space. Following a satisfactory placement, a transparent sterile dressing is applied over the catheter site, while the other length is secured with a plaster [15].

## 10. Drugs which are injected into the epidural space

Local anaesthetic agents are the most commonly used medications for epidural analgesia in the ICU. The commonest LA for epidural analgesia is plain bupivacaine, an amide which is approximately 95% protein bound and is metabolised primarily in the liver via conjugation with glucuronic acid [16]. It comes in three different concentrations: 0.25%, 0.5%, and 0.75%. Bupivacaine for use in the ICU for analgesia is the plain formulation (plain Marcaine), and it is usually administered via an epidural catheter either as intermittent boluses or as a continuous infusion. A dose of 10–15 mg may be administered bolus after a test dose as described above. The drug may be repeated PRN at 3–5 mg.

While administering epidural bupivacaine, monitoring for the motor block using the Modified Bromage scale [17] and watching out for local anaesthetic toxicity is necessary.

The scale is as follows:

| Score | Criteria |
|---|---|
| 1 | Complete block (unable to move feet or knees) |
| 2 | Almost complete block (able to move feet only) |
| 3 | Partial block (just able to move knees) |
| 4 | Detectable weakness of hip flexion while supine (full flexion of knees) |
| 5 | No detectable weakness of hip flexion while supine |
| 6 | Able to perform partial knee bend |

No block or partial block is desirable for ICU patients on epidural bupivacaine for pain relief.

Signs of local anaesthetic toxicity (LAST) may not be easily detectable in the sedated patient in the ICU, and thus, a high index of suspicion is required. Despite this, "the incidence of LAST in sedated patients is not higher than in others" [18].

Signs of LAST include:

- Light-headedness
- Agitation
- Tremor
- Tingling sensation around the mouth
- Convulsion
- Slurred speech
- Coma
- Cardiac arrest.

Early recognition and prompt intervention are advocated in order to prevent unfavourable outcomes.

Opioids are the main medications used for Analgesia in ICU patients due to their potency and a concomitant mild sedative and anxiolytic effects. It can be administered by multiple routes. The commonly used opioids include fentanyl, remifentanil, and morphine. Morphine is usually administered as a 2–5 mg bolus or at 1–20 mg/h via continuous infusion. Epidural administration of 5 mg of morphine sulphate can provide adequate postoperative [19] analgesia for up to 24 hours. Lower doses are however, recommended in patients with hepatic or renal insufficiency which is common among ICU patients.

One of the most common side effects of epidural morphine is respiratory depression, with an overall risk of less than 1%. This is nonetheless, similar to that of opioids administered via the parenteral route [20, 21]. Others are miosis, constipation, urinary retention, pruritus, hypotension, nausea and vomiting. The sedative effect of morphine is beneficial in patients in whom sedation is indicated, such as mechanically ventilated patients and those in whom invasive procedures need to be performed.

Other analgesic adjuvants may be administered via the epidural route to improve pain relief in critically ill patients in the ICU. These include α2-agonists, such as clonidine and dexmedetomidine. In addition to providing analgesia, dexmedetomidine infusion has been shown to reduce the prevalence and duration of confusion and delirium [22]. The side-effect profile of both α2-agonists includes bradycardia, cardiac asystole and hypotension. Although rare, it can cause rebound hypertension and can cause withdrawal syndrome [22].

## 11. Conclusion

Pain relief is an integral part of the management of critically ill patients in the intensive care unit. Epidural analgesia is a helpful component of a multimodal analgesia approach to patients in the ICU. Careful patient selection, availability of trained personnel and increased patient monitoring will ensure the safe delivery of epidural analgesia in the ICU.

## Author details

Kingsley U. Tobi
Faculty of Health Sciences and Veterinary Medicine, Department of Surgical Sciences, Division of Anaesthesiology, University of Namibia, Windhoek, Namibia

*Address all correspondence to: tobikingsley265@gmail.com

## References

[1] International Association for the Study of Pain (IASP) Taxonomy. Available from: http://www.iasp-pain.org/Education/Content.aspx?ItemNumber=1698&&navItemNumber=576

[2] de Jong A, Molinari N, De Lattre S. Decreasing severe pain and serious adverse events while moving intensive care unit patients: A prospective interventional study (the NURSE-DO project). Critical Care. 2013;**17**:R74

[3] Vazquez M, Pardavila MI, Lucia M, Aguado Y, Margall MA, Asiain MC. Pain assessment in turning procedures for patients with invasive mechanical ventilation. Nursing in Critical Care. 2011;**16**:178-185

[4] Granja C, Gomes E, Amaro A, et al. JMIP study group: Understanding post-traumatic stress disorder-related symptoms after critical care: The early illness amnesia hypothesis. Critical Care Medicine. 2008;**36**:2801-2809

[5] Marino PL. Analgesia and sedation. In: Marino PL, Sutin KM, editors. The ICU Book. 3rd ed. Philadelphia, PA: Lippincott Williams & Wilkins; 2007. pp. 885-907

[6] Akça O, Melischek M, Scheck T, et al. Postoperative pain and subcutaneous oxygen tension. Lancet. 1999;**354**:41-42

[7] Hedderich R, Ness TJ. Analgesia for trauma and burns. Critical Care Clinics. 1999;**15**:167-184

[8] Kirksey KM, McGlory G, Sefcik EF. Pain assessment and management in critically ill older adults. Critical Care Nursing Quarterly. 2015;**38**:237-244

[9] McGuire DB, Kaiser KS, Haisfield-Wolfe ME, Iyamu F. Pain assessment in non-communicative adult palliative care patients. The Nursing Clinics of North America. 2016;**51**:397-431

[10] Rijkenberg S, Stilma W, Endeman H, Bosman RJ, Oudemans-van Straaten HM. Pain measurement in mechanically ventilated critically ill patients: Behavioral pain scale versus critical-care pain observation tool. Journal of Critical Care. 2015;**30**:167-172

[11] Low JH. Survey of epidural analgesia management in general intensive care units in England. Acta Anaesthesiologica Scandinavica. 2002;**46**:799-805

[12] Schulz-Stübner S, Boezaart A, Hata S. Regional Analgesia in the critically ill. Critical Care Medicine. 2005;**33**:1400-1407

[13] Epidural management, Epidural Analgesia, Epidural Anesthesia, Thoracic. Available from: https://www.cancertherapyadvisor.com/home/decision-support-in-medicine/critical-care-medicine/epidural-management-epidural-analgesia-epidural-anesthesia-thoracic-epidural-lumbar-epidural-regional-anesthesia/

[14] Holladay J, Sage K. Epidural catheter. [Updated 2022 Jun 11]. In: StatPearls [Internet]. Treasure Island (FL): StatPearls Publishing; Jan 2022

[15] Gerheuser F, Roth A. Epidural anesthesia. Der Anaesthesist. 2007;**56**(5):499-523

[16] Bupivacaine HCL Injection and Bupivacaine and Epinephrine Injection. Available from: https://www.accessdata.fda.gov/drugsatfda_docs/label/2010/071165s020lbl.pdf

[17] Breen TW et al. Epidural anesthesia for labor in an ambulatory patient. Anesthesia and Analgesia. 1993;**77**:919-924

[18] Kessler P, Steinfeldt T, Gogarten W, Schwemmer U, Büttner J, Graf BM. Peripheral regional anesthesia in patients under general anesthesia: risk assessment with respect to parasthesia, injection pain and nerve damage. Der Anaesthesist. 2013;**62**(6):483-488

[19] Epidural Morphine Article—StatPearls. Available from: https://www.statpearls.com/articlelibrary/viewarticle/21231/

[20] Mugabure BB. A clinical approach to neuraxial morphine for the treatment of postoperative pain. Pain Research and Treatment. 2012;**2012**:612145

[21] Bujedo BM. Current evidence for spinal opioid selection in postoperative pain. The Journal of Pain. 2014;**27**(3):200-209

[22] Narayanan M, Venkataraju A, Jennings J. Analgesia in intensive care: part 1. BJA Education. 2016;**16**:72-78

Section 5

# Epidural Service and Low Resource Setting

Chapter 7

# Perspective Chapter: Epidural Anaesthesia Service Delivery in Anaesthesia Workforce Constrained Regions

*Chimaobi Tim Nnaji*

## Abstract

Epidural anaesthesia is often under-utilized in our environment. This could be linked to scarcity of specialist anaesthesia providers in anaesthesia workforce constrained regions. To have an effective and safe surgical and obstetric intervention, there is need to have specialist anaesthesia providers that proffer effective leadership in anaesthesia services and delivery of emergency and essential patient care, to help combat the extremely high avoidable anaesthesia-related morbidities and mortalities. Epidural anaesthesia can offer both intraoperative and postoperative analgesia, with the potential to reduce morbidity and mortality. It's use in labour analgesia has been found to be very effective, with good obstetric outcome. Nevertheless, epidural anaesthesia requires the availability of human, technical and economic resources. But, despite the fact that healthcare is given a strategic priority in the life of people, delivery of safe surgical and non-surgical services is linked to anaesthesia workforce capacity and its impact in the society.

**Keywords:** epidural anaesthesia, analgesia, specialist anaesthetist, anaesthesia workforce, safety

## 1. Introduction

Epidural anaesthesia and analgesia services is a technique for perioperative and procedural pain management with multiple applications that may be used as a primary surgical anaesthetic, resource for postoperative pain management, chronic pain relief or labour and obstetric delivery analgesia [1]. It is safe and relatively easy to perform by trained personnel. Nevertheless, it requires adequate training and high level of skill acquisition. Epidural anaesthesia and analgesia services takes into consideration the anatomy of the patient's spine, procedural indications and contraindications, in the view of the interprofessional teams' role in providing and improving care for patients who undergo surgery or require pain management. Irrespective of the benefit of potentially providing excellent analgesia, its use reduces the exposure of patient to other anaesthetics and analgesics, decreasing side effects [2]. Nevertheless, the importance of collaboration and communication amongst the health care team involved in the care of patients who receive epidural anaesthesia or analgesia service is important in improving outcomes. Epidural anaesthesia or analgesia can be administered as a single shot, intermittent/programmed bolus or a continuous infusion for long-term pain relief. Many beneficial aspects of epidural analgesia or anaesthesia have been reported, including better suppression of surgical and labour stress, positive effect on postoperative nitrogen balance, more stable cardiovascular haemodynamic, reduced blood loss, better peripheral vascular circulation, better labour analgesia and postoperative pain control [2].

Epidural anaesthesia and analgesia services is one of the unique facets of anaesthesia service delivery, which forms an important part of medical services in any country and undeniably strengthens the healthcare systems. Nevertheless, irrespective of the strategic priority given to healthcare in the life of the global population, the delivery of safe surgical and non-surgical services is linked to anaesthesia workforce capacity and its impact in the society. The epidural analgesia and anaesthesia services in any region of the world are particularly susceptible to the level of socio-economic development of such region, and like any other anaesthesia service delivery, the practice faces numerous challenges exclusively related to high number of pathologies, shortage of materials and drugs, infrastructure and human resources [3]. In many developing countries, especially sub-Saharan Africa, there is a critical shortage of healthcare workers and very limited resources. The health systems are stretched by diseases such as HIV/AIDS, tuberculosis, diarrhoea diseases and malaria and the loss of trained staff to the developed world and insecurities. Furthermore, economic effects of long-term conflict continue to rampage most of the developing countries.

Epidural anaesthesia and analgesia service are particularly vulnerable to development pressures and the quality of epidural anaesthesia and analgesia services is highly correlated with perioperative mortality and morbidity of the patients [4]. Hence, the presence of adequate infrastructure, skilled anaesthesia providers and the use of effective sanitation are paramount to improving the epidural anaesthesia and analgesia service, which will have a pro-founding positive effect on acute and chronic pain management services, obstetric services and perioperative outcome.

## 2. Shortage of physician anaesthesia specialist

Effective and safe pain care, surgical and obstetric intervention requires the presence of specialist anaesthesia providers that proffer quality leadership in epidural anaesthesia and analgesia services during elective, emergency and essential patient care, to help combat the extremely high avoidable anaesthesia-related morbidities and mortalities. This remains elusive in developing countries because of shortage of anaesthesia specialist among other healthcare workers [5, 6]. The number of surgical conditions contributing to the global burden of disease and the potential impact of such on basic surgical services continue to rise. It is estimated that 11% of the world's disability-adjusted life years are from conditions that are very likely to require surgery. Increasing evidence is beginning to emerge that maternal and infant survival is proportionately correlated to the number of health workers including physician anaesthetist providing obstetric care [5, 6]. Physician anaesthetists are scarce in many resource limited countries and they are not available at most referral health facilities and non-existent in remote and rural areas [3].

The number of Physician anaesthetists serving the looming population in the developing and resource limited countries has continued to decline irrespective of the soaring population, due to lack of political will, poor wages, conflicts and insecurities and migration to developed countries with better wage packages and incentives [3]. Mavalankar and coworkers [7], reported that in Afghanistan with population of 32 million persons, there are only 9 physician anaesthetists and only 8 in Bhutan with population less than 700,000. Another study observed that only 13 physician anaesthetist are available in Uganda to serve a surging population of 27 million persons [3]. Different studies conducted in Zimbabwe [8] and Nigeria [9, 10] identified that there are no specialist anaesthetists in public or provincial hospitals that serve as the referral centres in Zimbabwe and Nigeria respectively. World Health Organization (WHO) has encouraged member states to ensure that anaesthesia is properly prioritized within the health system and that support, follow-up, reporting, and bench-marking take place [11].

A report from the World Federation of Societies of Anaesthesiologist (WFSA) shows that there was a total of 436,596 physician anaesthesia provider in the 153 countries serving a population of more than 7 billion persons. This represents a workforce density of 6.09 per 100,000 population. The study also showed that 355,381 (81.4%) were specialist anaesthetists, 71,990 trainee specialist anaesthetists (16.5%), and 9225 (2.1%) non-specialist physician providers [12]. However, this figure is mainly dominated by developed country statistics. Most countries in Africa like Nigeria, Angola, Burkina Faso, Ethiopia, Zimbabwe and Niger has a workforce of <1 per 100,000 physician anaesthesia providers [12]. Indicating that resource limited and developing countries are still unable to meet the WFSA recommendation of at least 5 physician anaesthesia providers per 100,000 population, in other to ensure an effective leadership in anaesthesia services and delivery of emergency and essential patient care.

The scarcity of specialist anaesthesia physician can have a negative impact on the implementation of epidural anaesthesia and analgesia service in terms of the safety of perioperative, obstetric and pain patients, as well as the quality of healthcare services that will be delivered to the patients. The specialist anaesthesia physician in resource limited countries are over-worked irrespective of their limited number. For example, in Nigeria the physician anaesthetists in the public hospitals are involved in perioperative patient care, patient's resuscitation, critical care medicine, transportation of critically ill patients, acute and chronic pain management, sedation services, as well as healthcare system management, advocacy, simulation and medical education and research [13]. Furthermore, the private hospitals also depend on the services of this constrained specialist anaesthetists to sustain safe and quality healthcare services in their institutions. Thus, making them prone to burnouts and unable to sustain epidural anaesthesia and analgesia services.

## 3. Obstetrics epidural analgesia service challenges

Epidural analgesia is widely regarded as the gold standard for pain relief during labour. It involves the titration of low-dose and low-concentration local anaesthetics, to produce safe and reliable analgesia during labour and delivery. A properly monitored labour epidural service has a low incidence of side effects or serious complications to the parturient or foetus [14, 15]. However, in order for this service to be safe and efficacious, epidural labour analgesia need to be accessible 24 hours, every day. But the evaluation of this service in resource limited countries of the world shows that it is reluctantly or grossly low, or even not available in most health institutions that serves as referral healthcare facilities [16–18]. Furthermore, literature search on the utilization rate of epidural analgesia in labour in resource limited countries shows dearth of data in this region of the world, and it is associated with limited anaesthesia workforce, time constraint, limited anaesthesia materials and equipment, lack of advocacy and awareness of such service (see **Table 1**).

When Jacobs-Martin et al. [16] evaluated the utilization of epidural analgesia services in labour in South Africa women, they observed that the rate was abysmally low, with the incidence of 2.2%, compared with the rate of 23.4% and 90% in developed countries like United Kingdom and United State of America, respectively [24, 25]. They accrued the low rate of epidural analgesia in labour to limited number of available skilled anaesthesia personnel, time constraint, knowledgeable support staff, materials and equipment. Another study conducted by Okojie et al. [16] and Imaregiaye et al. [18] in Nigeria showed that the awareness of this service is grossly low, although with high level of acceptability among the educated and those with previous birth experience. Nevertheless, access to this service was very low, because of unavailability of 24 hours service as a result of low staff strength. In this region of the world, the ratio of physician anaesthesia provider is 0.58 per 100,000 population, instead of the recommended 5 per 100,000 population by WFSA [12]. This could be a determining factor to the lack of advocacy and effective epidural analgesia services in labour, as the limited available specialist anaesthetists are overwhelmed with perioperative and critical care services even at the referral health institutions.

Epidural analgesia is a technical procedure, performed under aseptic technique, where medications like local anaesthetics with or without an additive is injected into the epidural space with the intention of providing analgesia to a specific region of sensory dermatomes [26]. This is followed by subsequent intermittent or programmed top ups, until the mother delivers her baby in a pain free and safe scenario. The availability epidural analgesia service helps to conveys a level of safety to woman in labour and the foetus. Epidural analgesia service has traditionally been viewed as expensive, resource-intensive, time consuming and requiring highly specialized training for the doctors and support staff in resource limited clime. Thus, making it underutilized in this environment.

To deliver an effective and safe epidural analgesia service in labour, personnel, as well as some minimum equipment, materials and medications are required. This includes the availability of physician anaesthetist, obstetrician, trained nursing staff skilled with handling of epidural services and other support staff. There is also need for the availability of supplemental oxygen source, suction machine, related equipment, self-inflating bag and mask device that is able to provide positive pressure ventilation, airway materials like oropharyngeal airway, nasopharyngeal airway, endotracheal tubes for resuscitation, patient monitors with the capability for non-invasive blood pressure, electrocardiographic, pulse oximetry and capnographic monitoring. Furthermore, there is need to have intravenous catheters, crystalloids, infusion sets, syringes, needles, emergency drugs like vasopressors (ephedrine, phenylephrine, epinephrine), atropine, and intralipids, and defibrillators or crash cart [27].

The minimum equipment and medications required for obstetric epidural analgesia services are often not available in most health institutions in developing countries, making it difficult for the limited number of anaesthesia physicians to function and provide effective safe labour epidural analgesia services. The environment is associated with poor operation theatre infrastructure and unavailability of equipment,

| Author | Objective | Country | Findings | Conclusion |
|---|---|---|---|---|
| Fyneface-Ogan et al. [15] | To ascertain the outcome of labour and the views of multiparous Nigerian women in labour under epidural analgesia or parenteral opioids/ sedatives. | Nigeria | Epidural analgesia in labour offers 80% satisfaction and 8% inadequate analgesia in women in labour. | Epidural labour analgesia is acceptable to women in our setting, with high level of satisfaction with the experience of labour. |
| Jacobs-Martin et al. [16] | To establish the incidence of epidural analgesia in women in labour in a tertiary referral centre in the Western Cape | South Africa | Incidence of labour epidural analgesia was 2.2%, with complication rate of 32.3%. | Only 2.2% of women in labour received epidural analgesia, most likely because of time constraints on the limited available personnel. |
| Okojie et al. [17] | To assess the knowledge and perception of pregnant women regarding epidural analgesia for labour | Nigeria | About 79.5% of pregnant women are not aware of epidural analgesia service in labour. | There is poor awareness and acceptance of epidural analgesia in labour in this environment. |
| Imarengiaye et al. [18] | To determine the clinical correlates of the demand and utilization of labour analgesia resources by Nigerian women in labour | Nigeria | About 37.5% patients were aware that the pain of labour can be relieved but only 26.0% had prenatal information on labour analgesia. A total of 38.9%) did receive analgesia during labour. | There is poor utilization of labour analgesia services. |
| Leonard et al. [19] | To describe the labour epidural analgesia experience in a health institution in South Africa. | South Africa | Epidural analgesia in labour had an utilization rate of 1.6% and complication rate of 22.6%. | There is low incidence of labour epidural analgesia. |
| Ezeonu et al. [20] | To determine the awareness and utilization of epidural analgesia in labour in pregnant women Teaching Hospital. | Nigeria | About 43.3% of the patients were aware of epidural analgesia in labour, but only 7.5% had used it, with 95% satisfaction rate. | The knowledge and practice of epidural analgesia among parturients are low. |
| Nabukenya et al. [21] | To determine the knowledge, attitudes and use of labour analgesia among women attending the antenatal clinic. | Uganda | Only 7% of the participants had knowledge of labour analgesia, with only 20.9% of the fraction being aware of epidural analgesia in labour. Total of 79.2% of such women had their child birth in a national referral hospital. | There is a wide gap between the desire for labour analgesia and its availability. |

| Author | Objective | Country | Findings | Conclusion |
|---|---|---|---|---|
| Waldum et al. [22] | To assess disparities in the provision of epidural analgesia in planned vaginal birth according to maternal region of birth. | Sub-Saharan Africa | Primiparous women had epidural analgesia utilization rate of 33.8%, while the multiparous women had the rate of 9% for vaginal delivery respectively. | There are some disparities in the provision of epidural analgesia based on maternal birthplace. |
| Waldum et al. [22] | To assess disparities in the provision of epidural analgesia in planned vaginal birth according to maternal region of birth. | North Africa/ Middle East | Primiparous women had epidural analgesia utilization rate of 39.4%, while the multiparous women had the rate of 13.7% for vaginal delivery respectively. | There are some disparities in the provision of epidural analgesia based on maternal birthplace. |
| Waldum et al. [22] | To assess disparities in the provision of epidural analgesia in planned vaginal birth according to maternal region of birth. | East Asia/ Pacific | Primiparous women had epidural analgesia utilization rate of 31.0%, while the multiparous women had the rate of 11.2% for vaginal delivery respectively. | There are some disparities in the provision of epidural analgesia based on maternal birthplace. |
| Waldum et al. [22] | To assess disparities in the provision of epidural analgesia in planned vaginal birth according to maternal region of birth. | South Asia | Primiparous women had epidural analgesia utilization rate of 38.1%, while the multiparous women had the rate of 14.8% for vaginal delivery respectively. | There are some disparities in the provision of epidural analgesia based on maternal birthplace. |
| Ojiakor et al. [23] | To determine the rate of demand, indications, post-dural puncture headache rate and factors affecting demand for epidural analgesia among women in labour. | Nigeria | The demand for labour epidural in the study centre was low with a demand rate of 2.6% | The demand for labour epidural analgesia in the study was low and there is a need for an enhanced awareness programs on obstetrics epidural analgesia. |

**Table 1.**
*Global epidural anaesthesia and analgesia indices and characteristics.*

lifesaving drugs and anaesthetic agents [3, 28]. Furthermore, the physicians face problems of unreliable electricity, unavailability of compressed oxygen and other gases, sophisticated machines and modern drugs [3, 28]. Safe provision of labour epidural analgesia service necessitates the ability to manage any potential complications or emergencies that may arise. There should be resuscitative equipment and drugs in the event of bradycardia, hypotension, high or total spinal anaesthesia, local anaesthetic toxicity or cardiopulmonary arrest, but these are either not available or in limited supplies.

The development of an epidural analgesia service should encompass patients' safety as part of its working protocols. Although the barriers to safe and effective administration of labour analgesia service like inadequate practitioner training, staff reserves, and unavailability of the proper technologies and medicines continue to rampage low resource countries, the desire for such services appears to exist, with evidence that when it is offered, some women chose to accept the service [16, 24].

## 4. Epidural anaesthesia service for surgeries and safety challenges

Epidural anaesthesia involves the injection of high volume and dose of local anaesthetic agent into the epidural space to achieve a reversible loss of sensation adequate to allow surgical procedures. It is usually administered for surgeries in the lower abdomen, perineum and lower extremities. Studies have shown that thoracic epidural anaesthesia can be used to perform major upper abdominal and thoracic surgeries, including cardiac and major thoracic vascular surgeries [29, 30]. Although epidural anaesthesia onset of action is slow, and sometimes associated with patchy sensory blocks, when properly performed, it can offer good anaesthesia and outlast the duration of prolonged surgeries. Nevertheless, the epidural anaesthetic effect on reducing intraoperative and postoperative morbidity and mortality varies with the type of surgery performed. Epidural anaesthesia can be performed as a sole anaesthetic or in combination with spinal or general anaesthesia. Its duration of anaesthesia is prolonged with the use of epidural catheters that allows for top ups or continuous injections of local anaesthetic and mixture with additive or local anaesthetic alone, to improve the overall surgical outcome. When used for abdominal aortic surgery, it can shorten the intubation time and intensive care stay [15, 31].

Epidural anaesthesia service requires the availability of human, technical and economic resources. In the present clime of patient safety, people in developing countries continue to suffer due to lack of trained physician anaesthetists, as well as lack of adequate health system infrastructure and equipment, prioritization of anaesthesia and surgical care as part of national health plans. The crisis in human resources for anaesthesia care in many developing countries is contributed by the low standing of the profession, especially in sub-Saharan Africa, and the resulting problems with recruitment and retention of practitioners at all levels. Hence, making it difficult for majority of the population in resource limited areas to access safe anaesthesia services both in cities and in the rural and underprivileged areas of the region. Safe surgical and non-surgical services is a reflection of adequate anaesthesia workforce capacity. Hence, improvements in the safety and quality of anaesthesia is urgently needed, but the challenge is the deficiency in the number of trained physician anaesthetist [32, 33].

Epidural anaesthesia is often under-utilized in our environment. This could be linked to scarcity of specialist anaesthesia providers in anaesthesia workforce constrained regions. To provide guidance and assistance in maintaining and improving the quality and safety of epidural anaesthesia service, specialist physician anaesthesia providers are required. The shortage of specialist anaesthesia physician creates a major hindrance and vacuum for epidural anaesthesia services in the resource limited areas of the world. In some countries, the gap is filled by non-physician anaesthetists, who provides any form of anaesthesia for surgical procedures. Most times they work alone without any support from specialist physician anaesthetists, and they handle cases beyond their training, with the number of morbidity and mortality relating to inappropriate care rising [34, 35]. Pignaton and colleagues reported that the quality of anaesthesia services delivered is highly correlated with perioperative morbidity and mortality [34]. A study showed that the overall risk of maternal death when non-physician anaesthetists provided care was 9.8 per 1000 compared to 5.2 per 1000 in physician anaesthesia provider care [35].

A meta-analytical study on anaesthesia related maternal mortality in low-income and middle-income countries, shows that in women undergoing an obstetric procedure, the risk of death attributed to anaesthesia was 1·2 per 1000 women, with the highest rates of 1·5 per 1000 in sub-Saharan Africa women. Anaesthesia was reported as the main cause of death in 2.8% of all direct and indirect maternal deaths, with the highest rates in Middle East and North Africa (6.2%), and the lowest in east Asia and Pacific (1.5%). When neuraxial anaesthesia like epidural anaesthesia were compared with the administration of general anaesthesia, the odds of maternal death tripled, with mortality rates of 5.9 per 1000 in general anaesthesia and 1.2 per 1000 for neuraxial anaesthesia. General anaesthesia also doubled the odds of perinatal death compared with neuraxial block [35]. Availability of specialist anaesthesia physician in the resource limited regions will be effective in ensuring leadership in epidural anaesthesia services, delivery of obstetric emergencies and essential patient care. Epidural anaesthesia service use in obstetrics has been found to be very effective, with good obstetric outcome. Epidural anaesthesia service can provide safe and efficient anaesthesia for unplanned or emergent Caesarean delivery by increasing the dose and concentration of the local anaesthetics and/or the adjuvant used for labour analgesia [15, 27].

To ensure safety of lives and improve perioperative care, modern anaesthesia practice has become increasingly dependent on complex equipment and expensive drugs, but this is only obtainable in high income countries. The resource limited regions and countries depend on basic equipment and essential drugs, however, in most places even the basic anaesthesia equipment and essential drugs are not available. Hence, limiting the practice of epidural anaesthesia.

## 5. Conclusion

Epidural anaesthesia and analgesia service is required for safe surgical and non-surgical ministration. It provides both intraoperative and postoperative analgesia and reduces perioperative morbidity and mortality. A properly monitored labour epidural service has a low incidence of side effects or serious complications to the parturient or foetus. But this service is often under-utilized in the workforce constrained developing and resource limited countries due to scarcity of specialist anaesthesia providers, as well as unavailability of infrastructural, technical and economic resources. Hence, to achieve an effective and sustainable epidural anaesthesia and analgesia service, there is need to increase and ensure the presence of adequate infrastructure, materials and resources and skilled anaesthesia providers. Resolution of the human resource crisis for anaesthesia care in many developing and limited resource countries will require the commitment of the government and high level of political will, to facilitate the recruitment and retention of specialist physician anaesthesia practitioners and their support staff at all levels of the healthcare system.

## Acknowledgements

I will like to express my deepest appreciation to God for his wisdom and to all the authors, whose work formed the foundation for this medical writing.

No funding was received for this work.

## Conflict of interest

The authors declare no conflict of interest.

## Author details

Chimaobi Tim Nnaji
Department of Anaesthesia, Federal Medical Centre, Owerri, Imo State, Nigeria

*Address all correspondence to: chymaoby@yahoo.com

## References

[1] Avila Hernandez AN, Singh P. Epidural Anesthesia. Treasure Island (FL): StatPearls Publishing; 2022. Available from: https://www.ncbi.nlm.nih.gov/books/NBK542219/?report=classic. [Updated March 9, 2022]

[2] Rodgers A, Walker N, Schug S, et al. Reduction of postoperative mortality and morbidity with epidural or spinal anaesthesia: Results from overview of randomised trials. British Medical Journal. 2000;**321**:1493-1497

[3] Hodges SC, Mijumbi C, Okello M, McCormick BA, Walker IA, Wilson IH. Anaesthesia services in developing countries: Defining the problems. Anaesthesia. 2007;**62**:4-11

[4] Park WY, Thompson JS, Lee KK. Effect of epidural anesthesia and analgesia on perioperative outcome: A randomized, controlled veterans affairs cooperative study. Annals of Surgery. 2001;**234**(4):560-571. DOI: 10.1097/00000658-200110000-00015 PMID: 11573049; PMCID: PMC1422079

[5] World Alliance for Patient Safety. WHO guidelines for safe surgery. Geneva: World Health Organization; 2008 [Accessed 02 Sep 2022]

[6] Robinson JJ, Wharrad H. The relationship between attendance at birth and maternal mortality rates: An exploration of United Nations' data sets including the ratios of physicians and nurses to population, GNP per capita and female literacy. Journal of Advanced Nursing. 2001;**34**:445-455. DOI: 10.1046/j.1365- 2648.2001.01773.x PMID:11380711

[7] Mavalankar D, Sriram V. Provision of anaesthesia services for emergency obstetric care through task shifting in South Asia. Reproductive Health Matters. 2009;**17**:21-31. DOI: 10.1016/S0968-8080(09)33433-3 PMID:19523579

[8] Lonnée HA, Madzimbamuto F, Erlandsen ORM, Vassenden A, Chikumba E, Dimba R, et al. Anesthesia for cesarean delivery: A cross-sectional survey of provincial, district, and Mission hospitals in Zimbabwe. Anesthesia and Analgesia. 2018;**126**(6):2056-2064. DOI: 10.1213/ANE.0000000000002733 PMID: 29293184

[9] Nuhu SI, Embu HY, Onoja AA, Dung D. Anaesthesia workforce and infrastructure in a north central state of Nigeria: A survey. Highland Medical Research Journal. 2017;**17**(1): 50-54

[10] Kalu QN, Eshiet AI, Ukpabio EI, Etiuma AU, Monjok E. A rapid need assessment survey of Anaesthesia and surgical Services in District Public Hospitals in Cross River state, Nigeria. British Journal of Medical Practitioners. 2014;**7**(4):a733

[11] The World Health report 2014. Strengthening emergency and essential surgical care and anaesthesia as a component of universal health coverage. Geneva: World Health Organization; 2014. Available from: http://apps.who.int/gb/ebwha/pdf_files/WHA68/A68_31-en.pdf [Accessed 14 Mar 2022]

[12] Kempthorne P, Morriss WW, Mellin-Olsen J, Gore-Booth J. The WFSA global anesthesia workforce survey. Anesthesia and Analgesia. 2017;**125**(3):981-990. DOI: 10.1213/ANE.0000000000002258 PMID: 28753173

[13] Nnaji CT. This medical field called Anaesthesia. Gazette Med. 2013;**1**(2):65-66

[14] Leighton BL, Halpern SH. The effects of epidural analgesia on labour, maternal, and neonatal outcomes: A systematic review. American Journal of Obstetrics and Gynecology. 2002;**186**(5):69-77

[15] Fyneface-Ogan S, Mato CN, Anya SE. Epidural anesthesia: Views and outcomes of women in labor in a Nigerian hospital. Annals of African Medicine. 2009;**8**(4):250-256

[16] Jacobs-Martin GG, Burke JL, Levin AI, Coetzee AR. Labour epidural analgesia audit in a teaching hospital in a developing country. Southern African Journal of Anaesthesia and Analgesia. 2014;**20**(4):174-178

[17] Okojie NQ, Isah EC. Perception of epidural analgesia for labour among pregnant women in a Nigerian tertiary hospital setting. Journal of the West African College of Surgeons. 2014;**4**(4):142

[18] Imarengiaye C, Ande A. Demand and utilisation of labour anal- gesia service by Nigerian women. Journal of Obstetrics and Gynaecology. 2006;**26**:130-132

[19] Leonard T, Perrie H, Scribante J, Chetty S. An audit of the labour epidural analgesia service at a regional hospital in Gauteng Province, South Africa. South African Journal of Obstetrics and Gynaecology. 2018;**24**(2):52-56

[20] Ezeonu PO, Anozie OB, Onu FA, Esike CU, Mamah JE, Lawani LO, et al. Perceptions and practice of epidural analgesia among women attending antenatal clinic in FETHA. International Journal of Women's Health. 2017;**9**:905-911

[21] Nabukenya MT, Kintu A, Wabule A, Muyingo MT, Kwizera A. Knowledge, attitudes and use of labour analgesia among women at a low-income country antenatal clinic. BMC Anesthesiology. 2015;**15**:98

[22] Waldum ÅH, Jacobsen AF, Lukasse M, Staff AC, Falk RS, Vangen S, et al. The provision of epidural analgesia during labor according to maternal birthplace: A Norwegian register study. BMC Pregnancy and Childbirth. 2020;**20**(1):321. DOI: 10.1186/s12884-020-03021-8 PMID: 32456615; PMCID: PMC7249666

[23] Ojiakor SC, Obidike AB, Okeke KN, Nnamani CP, Obi-Nwosu AL, et al. Factors associated with demand for epidural analgesia among women in labor at a tertiary hospital in Nnewi, south-east, Nigeria. Magna Scientia Advanced Research and Reviews. 2021;**02**(01):008-013. DOI: 10.30574/msarr.2021.2.1.0028

[24] The Office for National Statistics. Review of the National Statistician on Births and Patterns of Family Building in England and Wales, 2007. England and Wales: A National Statistics Publication; 2008 [Accessed 10 Aug 2022]

[25] Wong CA. Advances in labor analgesia. International Journal of Women's Health. 2009;**10**(1):139-154

[26] Silva M, Halpern SH. Epidural analgesia for labour: Current techniques. Local and Regional Anesthesia. 2010;**3**:143-153

[27] Kodali BS, Jagannathan DK, Owen MD. Establishing an obstetric neuraxial service in low-resource areas. International Journal of Obstetric Anesthesia. 2014;**23**(3):267-273

[28] Petroze RT, Nzayisenga A, Rusanganwa V, et al. Comprehensive national analysis of emergency and

essential surgical capacity in Rwanda. The British Journal of Surgery. 2012;**99**:436-443

[29] McLeod GA, Cumming C. Thoracic epidural anaesthesia and analgesia. Continuing Education in Anaesthesia, Critical Care and Pain. 2004;**4**(1):16-19. DOI: 10.1093/bjaceaccp/mkh006

[30] Svircevic V, Nierich AP, Moons KGM, Diephuis JC, Ennema JJ, et al. Thoracic epidural anesthesia for cardiac surgery: A randomized trial. Anesthesiology. 2011;**114**:262-270. DOI: 10.1097/ALN.0b013e318201d2de

[31] Parkin IG, Harrison GR. The topographical anatomy of the lumbar epidural space. Journal of Anatomy. 1985;**141**:211-217

[32] Meara JG, Leather AJM, Hagander L, Alkire BC, Alonso N, Ameh EA, et al. Global surgery 2030: Evidence and solutions for achieving health, welfare, and economic development. Lancet. 2015;**386**:569-624

[33] Hansen D, Gausi SC, Merikebu M. Anaesthesia in Malawi: Complications and deaths. Tropical Doctor. 2000;**30**:146-149

[34] Pignaton W, Braz JR, Kusano PS, Módolo MP, de Carvalho LR, Braz MG, et al. Perioperative and anesthesia-related mortality: An 8-year observational survey from a tertiary teaching hospital. Medicine (Baltimore). 2016;**95**(2):e2208

[35] Sobhy S, Zamora J, Dharmarajah K, Arroyo-Manzano D, Wilson M, et al. Anaesthesia-related maternal mortality in low-income and middle-income countries: A systematic review and meta-analysis. The Lancet Global Health. 2016;**4**:e320-e327